Hidden in Plain Sight

A Guidebook for How to Stop Teen Vaping

Hidden in Plain Sight

A Guidebook for How to Stop Teen Vaping

By Lauren Ibekwe, MPH, ACPS, & Payal Patani, ACPS, with Fort Bend Regional Council/Fort Bend Community Prevention Coalition, & Uzo Odili, MD, Medical Director for APEX Urgent Care

Preface

Before, I was blind. Now, I see the truth. When vaping devices were first announced as a potential mechanism to help cigarette smokers quit smoking, I was hopeful. I knew that the rate of smoking in teens and adults were both falling year after year for decades. I wanted to see the end of cigarette smoking and all the associated health consequences, so I wanted to believe the hype. I didn't know that the tobacco companies were looking for a way to acquire new customers to replace the people who were quitting cigarettes. I didn't know that they would engineer a new form of nicotine that absorbed into the body and affected the brain faster than the nicotine in cigarettes. I didn't know that they would primarily manufacture the products in fruity flavors and aim their marketing algorithms at teens and young adults. I didn't know that drug dealers would modify vape juice by adding THC and other drugs to make a harmful habit into a deadly one. I didn't know that the product they described as a solution would become one of the biggest problems threatening the health of our teens today. But now that I know these things, I need all of you to know them too. This book is for every concerned parent, teacher, neighbor, aunt, uncle, grandparent, and friend who knows someone who vapes and doesn't know what to say to convince him or her to stop. I dedicate this book to you, and I hope that it helps you and your loved ones.

Table of Contents

TESTIMONIALS FROM PARENTS WHO HAVE LEARNED FROM THE HIDDEN IN PLAIN SIGHT PRESENTATIONS

"Room decor, obscure compartments, and items to camouflage located throughout the room provide red flags and potential warning signs for parents of how teens may hide alcohol, drugs, and vaping products. Parents must take meaningful steps to address a young person's use and change the quality of a young teen for a positive change".

- Dimpy Koul, FBISD Parent and Associate Professor, Brain Tumor Center, MD Anderson Cancer Center

"The bedroom is illuminating. It's amazing to see how these devices have changed over the past 30 years. It's a testament to why we do the work we do."

- Ray Andrews, Director of Houston Crackdown-Office of the Mayor

"The Hidden in Plain Sight bedroom is an eye-opening experience for anyone who gets the opportunity to see it. It allows you to see the deception and ingenuity of a drug user."

- Dawn Mathis, Public Affairs Specialist, Drug Enforcement Agency, Houston Division

INTRODUCTION

As a physician and a parent, I know that you have questions about vaping. You've probably seen vaping devices on social media and in movies, where they depict vaping as a safe recreational activity. They'll make it look cool and safe, but they won't tell you about the risk of nicotine addiction or the risks associated with inhaling dangerous chemicals. This comprehensive guide was designed to answer all of your questions on vaping and more. It will educate you about the science that proves the danger is real.

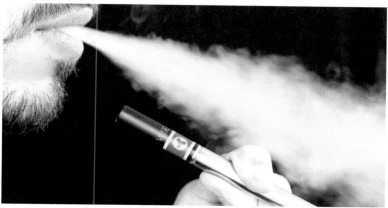

A Vuse vape pen in a sleek silver and black finish makes a dangerous activity look interestingly attractive.

The struggle to end teen vaping is an uphill battle. The billion-dollar corporations who own the vaping companies fill the airwaves and internet with advertising that makes vaping seem safe and cool. Our teens are being conditioned to think that vaping is a recreational activity with no risk, but this is so far from the truth it is almost embarrassing.

School principals tell me that even elementary school kids are bringing vaping devices to school now. You could not imagine 10-year-olds smoking cigarettes or drinking liquor, but somehow, they can access vaping devices. This can only happen in an environment where parents do not know the risk of vaping. I believe that the best action we can take to prevent teen vaping is to educate parents about the dangers of vaping and nicotine.

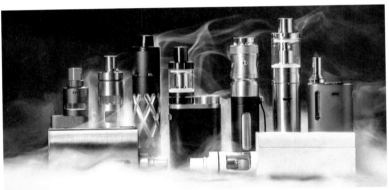

A collection of modern vaping devices. Their stylish appearances are geared toward attracting modern young new users.

This guide contains a review of the latest clinical research and national surveys to provide the most accurate information. More importantly, we break it down into plain language so that you and your teens (or young adults) will all be able to understand why vaping is such a dangerous activity. We have spent the past five years educating the public at high school auditoriums, community events, and town hall gatherings. After speaking with thousands of concerned parents, teachers, students, and school nurses about the teen vaping epidemic, we are confident that this guide will answer all your questions.

The vaping epidemic is real. Since 2011, the US Food and Drug Administration (FDA) and the Centers for Disease Control (CDC) have surveyed middle and high school students annually to find out how common youth tobacco abuse really is. Traditional cigarette use in kids had been decreasing every year for several years, but the new data suggested that the trends were reversing. In 2014, e-cigarette use became the leading method of tobacco abuse in kids, surpassing traditional cigarette use.

Although vaping was initially introduced in America as an alternate method for current cigarette smokers to attempt to quit smoking, electronic cigarettes never got FDA approval for that purpose. Instead, vaping companies began advertising to young people with flashy ads and nightlife events with free samples. Vaping has become a recreational activity and the leading vehicle by which teenagers are introduced to tobacco and nicotine.

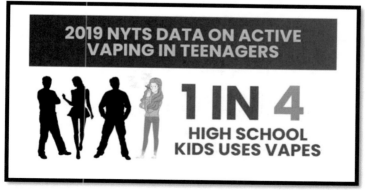

The 2019 National Youth Tobacco Survey (NYTS), a large-scale survey of teens conducted by the CDC and FDA, reported that over five million students indicated they had used e-cigarettes within the past 30 days and that 1 million of those students use them daily. This means that 1 in 4 high school students and 1 in 10 middle school students is vaping casually or on a regular basis.

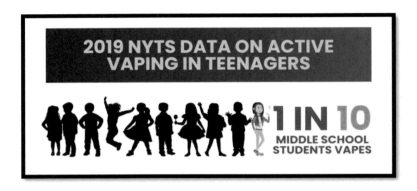

In 2020, we first learned about e-cigarette and vaping associated lung injury (EVALI), a mysterious pattern of lung disease that seemed to mostly affect young people who vaped. Many people died, and the news media made vaping the center of attention for several weeks.

The NYTS results from the 2020 survey indicated about 3.6 million US middle and high school students self-reported some type of electronic cigarette use within the previous 30 days. This was a significant drop from the previous year, but researchers could not pinpoint the factor with the greatest impact on the decrease in teen vaping. Active campaigns to educate teens on vaping risks and general fear of EVALI likely both contributed to the decline.

Details from the survey revealed that use of refillable pods decreased, and use of disposable e-cigarettes increased in comparison to 2019 results. Among high school students, the self-reported use of disposable e-cigarettes increased from 2.4% to 26.5%, which coincided with new products emerging in the marketplace and increased spending on e-cigarette marketing. Refillable pods allowed users to customize the contents of e-liquid, providing the opportunity to even add other drugs to the mix. Disposable e-cigarettes are sealed by the manufacturer, preventing tampering, but they were offered in attractive, new fruity flavors. Around the same time, the FDA banned most vape juice flavors in refillable format, but not flavored one-time use vaping devices.

Further research also showed that big tobacco companies and e-cigarette startups used social media platforms like Twitter, Instagram, TikTok, and YouTube to market specifically to teens. These same studies showed a timely correlation between higher levels of marketing spending, a rise in the rate of youth nicotine abuse, and an increase in business profit[i]. We will discuss the relationship between marketing and vaping in more detail in another chapter.

In 2021, the COVID-19 pandemic was a life-changing event for everyone, and it significantly impacted the way the NYTS survey was conducted. During that time, many schools transitioned online, and the primary vehicle for social interaction between kids who vaped and kids who didn't was temporarily halted. Amid widespread school closures, the typical method of interviewing students in person to obtain accurate data also had to transition to a virtual version. Researchers were no longer able to visit with kids on campus, forcing them to only collect data online. Millions of students also stopped attending school in person and may not have been notified about the survey. Because of these changes, we cannot directly compare 2021 results to data from 2020 and prior years.

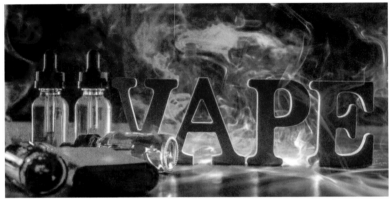

Another vaping advertisement promoting mystery and intrigue while hiding the drug's dangerous truths.

The 2021 NYTS survey indicated that two million middle and high school students reported e-cigarette use at least once in the previous 30 days. Among high school students who admitted to vaping, nearly 45% reported at least every-other-day use and 27.6% reported daily use[ii]. The survey allowed students to indicate their e-cigarette brand of choice with the following results: 26.1% of high school students indicated Puff Bar was their usual brand, 10.8% reported Vuse, 9.6% preferred SMOK, and 5.7% chose JUUL. 15.6% of high school users reported not knowing what brand they used. Among middle school users, 30.3% reported their regular brand was Puff Bar, 12.5% preferred JUUL, and 19.3% indicated not knowing the brand they used regularly[iii]. Among all users of all types of e-cigarettes (disposables, cartridge or pod type, or refillable tanks) the top flavors reported were fruit, followed by candy, desserts, or other sweets.

The NYTS survey conducted in 2022 revealed that 16.5% of high school students indicated they used a tobacco product within the previous 30 days[iv]. In other words, if your teenage child invited over six friends, one of those friends may have used a tobacco product in the previous month. 14% of high school students specifically indicated vaping as their tobacco delivery vehicle, meaning that one in seven high school kids is vaping actively. For middle school children, the rate of kids using tobacco products was 1 in 21 children, slightly less than 5%.

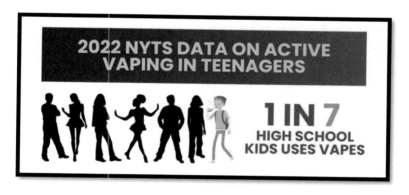

Over three million children in the survey admitted to tobacco use in the previous month, and two out of every three teenage tobacco users reported electronic cigarettes or vape devices as the nicotine delivery device they used on a regular basis. Over 80% of the kids who used e-cigarettes reported using products with flavors such as fruit, candy, or dessert-themed nicotine products, which are not as commonly used by adults.

7

Parents who want to actively protect their children from the risks of vaping and the lifelong effects of nicotine addiction must first arm themselves with knowledge about vaping and nicotine. We lay the groundwork for your success by using a physician's expertise to make sense of the latest reports from the CDC and the current research around the world. This guide summarizes that information in easy-to-digest question and answer segments. Our goal is to give you the tools you need to engage your teenagers (and anyone else) in healthy discussion on the risks and consequences of vaping.

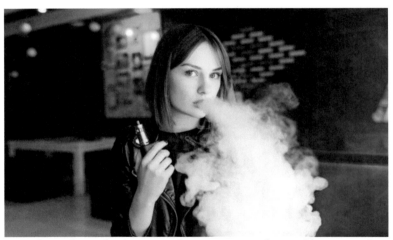

Vaping ads prefer images of younger people smoking to make vaping seem more acceptable to youth.

Chapter 1

WHAT IS VAPING AND WHY IS IT SO DANGEROUS?

Before you start an important conversation, it's good to make sure you have the vocabulary down so that you and your child are speaking the same language.

What is vaping?

Vaping, also called "Juuling," refers to the use of an electronic cigarette to aerosolize a chemical solution that contains nicotine or marijuana or both, and then inhale those drugs and chemicals. Vaping is neither safe, nor healthy. Vaping is now mostly a recreational activity, which means most manufacturers are not claiming any approved medical benefit and users are not intending to receive any medical benefit.

Vaping is also a clever and deceptive marketing tool to rebrand a dangerous activity to look like a safe activity. Vaping devices heat chemicals until they become tiny particles that suspend in the air so that the user can inhale them. The term "vaping" silently suggests the products are water-based and that steam or water vapor is what comes out, but vaping is much more like traditional cigarette smoking than most people think.

What is an electronic cigarette (e-cigarette)?

The electronic cigarette is a small device that uses energy from a rechargeable or disposable battery to activate a heating element to convert liquid nicotine to an aerosol, which is smoke filled with floating chemicals. The heating element is called an atomizer or a clearomizer. A clearomizer is a combination of an atomizer and an e-liquid reservoir. Of note, vaping devices are not allowed in checked luggage of airplanes because of the risk of battery or device explosion.

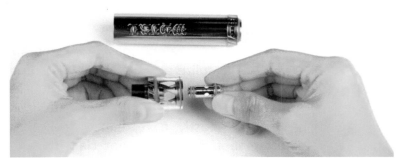

A vaping device deconstructed ... the heating element and the battery power source are shown here.

The devices are also called "vape pen," "Juul," or "puffbar." Newer models offer larger e-liquid reservoirs and the ability to regulate temperature and voltage. Some use disposable cartridges and others use refillable cartridges. These new levels of customization only make vaping more dangerous, as higher doses of nicotine and toxins within the aerosol are inhaled when using the larger devices.

10

What is an electronic nicotine delivery system (ENDS)?

To make it easier to classify and control the wide variety of vapes, vaporizers, vape pens, and hookah pens, the government developed a new classification name – electronic nicotine delivery system or ENDS for short. Traditional electronic cigarettes, e-cigs, and e-pipes also fall under this category. The government prefers to not use the term "vaping" because of the confusing nature of the term suggesting that only water vapor is being released instead of smoke and chemicals.

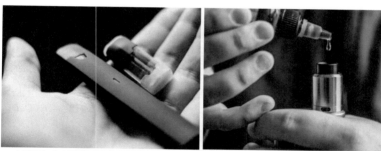

LEFT: A USB-style vape pen and a disposable vape cartridge. RIGHT: A vape juice dropper adding vape juice into the atomizer cartridge of a refillable vaping device.

What is vape juice?

It is important to highlight that e-liquid is not pure water inside a vape pen, Juul pod, or any other electronic cigarette. Equally important is the fact that vape juice is not juice at all. These terms were intentionally chosen to mislead users into thinking that vaping products are more healthy than traditional cigarettes.

Vape juice, or e-liquid, is an oil-based chemical liquid that

11

aerosolizes when heated by the e-cigarette. The chemical mixture usually contains liquid nicotine, water, flavoring, and either a propylene glycol or vegetable glycerin base. The liquid contents of a vaping cartridge are not food and should never be tasted, swallowed, or ingested in any way. The nicotine and the flavoring chemicals are dissolved into the other components so that they do not settle at the bottom like the pulp you see in a bottle of orange juice. There are some versions that allow the user to mix ingredients and add their own flavoring to the liquid nicotine mixture.

Normally, you would look at an ingredients label to learn if an item is good for your health. Unfortunately, with vaping liquids, the ingredients listed can be intentionally misleading, or it may contain the list of chemicals present at room temperature, not the chemicals that form once the liquid is heated and the components become aerosolized.

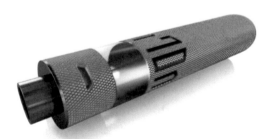

A vape pen designed to camouflage as a USB flash drive.

What is a vape mod?

A vape mod, or mechanical vape mod, is a newer form of

electronic cigarette with a larger size and usually a more powerful battery. The increased power allows the vape juice to heat to higher temperatures which produces more aerosol or smoke than standard vape pens. Companies advertise this as getting more flavor, although more aerosol also means more hazardous elements. Users also have the option to add extra components to the vape juice which can increase the risk of harm from ingesting unknown substances even further.

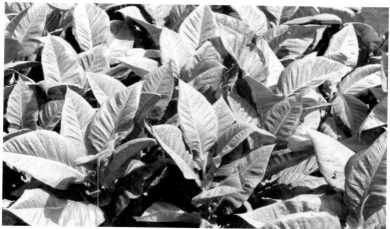

A collection of natural tobacco plants. You'd never imagine such an addictive drug was hiding inside this bush.

What is nicotine?

Nicotine is a natural compound found in tobacco plants that acts as a stimulant for the brain. When nicotine reaches the brain, dopamine levels increase, which causes a temporary sensation of pleasure and relaxation. This pleasing feeling of well-being is part of why nicotine is so addictive. Nicotine use also triggers the release of adrenalin, also known as epinephrine, which causes an increase in heart rate and blood pressure. The half-life of nicotine is about 2 hours, which means nearly all of the nicotine that enters your body will be gone in 8-10 hours. When nicotine is broken down by the body, it becomes cotinine, a non-addictive byproduct of nicotine that does not create the same effects on the body. Cotinine lasts much longer in the body and drug testing measures the level of cotinine as a way of looking for nicotine use.

When a cigarette is burned and consumed, the nicotine and other dry ingredients become tiny particles suspended in smoke. Nicotine inhaled from cigarette smoke causes users to experience a burning sensation and irritation in the back of the throat. Tobacco companies countered this fact by adding menthol to cigarettes to cool the tongue and throat. Some tobacco manufacturers also added lidocaine, a numbing agent used by dentists and doctors, to their cigarette products to reduce the burning sensation.

What is propylene glycol?

Propylene glycol is a synthetic liquid that the FDA considers "generally safe" in food, cosmetics, and pharmaceutical drugs. Propylene glycol is used in foods to maintain moisture and preserve flavor in prepared foods. You can find propylene glycol in vanilla extract, almond extract, and other food coloring or flavorings.

However, research has shown that inhalation of propylene glycol caused significant irritation of the throat and upper airway.[v] Furthermore, when propylene glycol is heated, it converts partially to propylene oxide and formaldehyde, which are both known carcinogens. This means people who are repeatedly exposed to these chemicals have developed certain cancers in higher rates than the general public.[vi]

What is vegetable glycerin?

Vegetable glycerin is a sugary alcohol derived from plant oils. It is typically colorless and odorless. The FDA classifies it as "generally safe" for consumption, but this designation does not apply to inhalation of the compound in a vapor or aerosol form. Interestingly, both propylene glycol and vegetable glycerin are both commonly used to create vapor, smoke, and fog for stage performances in the entertainment industry.

When glycerin is heated, it partially converts to the compound acrolein, a potent pulmonary irritant and carcinogen[vii]. This means acrolein damages the lungs and can increase your chances of developing cancer. A study of employees with regular exposure to these fogs showed they suffered an increase in respiratory problems.[viii] Short-term exposure led to dry throat and coughing, while long-term exposure was associated with chronic wheezing and chest tightness.

Acrolein is also one of the harmful chemicals that was found in higher levels than normal after the train derailment and chemical spill in the state of Ohio in February of 2023. Acrolein was not being transported on the train, but it can be formed by combustion of the chemicals that were transported on the train that derailed.

Does an e-cigarette release smoke like a cigarette?

When an electronic cigarette heats up e-liquid, many chemical reactions occur that release hazardous elements in the form of an aerosol or smoke. Even though e-cigarettes do not burn tobacco, they still release harmful chemicals in breathable form. Several compounds that increase the risk of developing cancer have been identified in the aerosol from vaping devices. Flavor additives like diacetyl and 2,3-pentanedione can convert to carcinogenic chemicals when heated, forming acrolein, propylene oxide, and acrylamide.

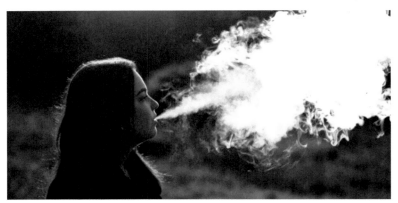

Teens start vaping for different reasons but become addicted due to nicotine. Performing vape smoke tricks is a secondary recreational benefit that keeps some vapers entertained.

The wires that transfer energy from the battery to the atomizer and the filament that holds the heat can be made of copper, tin, nickel, chromium, silica, silver, and iron. Inhaling these chemicals and metals causes damage to the lungs, and in some cases, the damage is irreversible. Researchers have analyzed the aerosol output from

16

several different types of vape pens and vape mods and found the presence of these same metals in higher concentrations than what would be in an equivalent amount of traditional cigarette smoke.[ix] Certain metals that are considered essential minerals, such as iron, nickel, and chromium, are safe to eat. However, inhaling them deeply is quite dangerous. Inhalation of silica particles or silica dust causes inflammation damage to the lung tissue. This can lead to a chronic respiratory disease called silicosis that cannot be cured. This means that repeated vape pen use can damage your lungs permanently.

What are THC and CBD? Are they related to vaping lung problems and vaping deaths?

Marijuana, also called cannabis, has been legal in most states in some form or another. Hemp is a variety of the cannabis plant. The 2018 Farm Bill allowed for all 50 states to legalize hemp farming as well as the production, sale, and widespread use of hemp. All forms of marijuana contain dozens of plant compounds called terpenes, but tetrahydrocannabinol, or THC for short, is the only component that has a long history of getting people "high". Cannabidiol or CBD is another compound that is extracted from the cannabis plant, but CBD does not have a psychoactive effect, so using it does not lead to a high. Emerging research suggests many medical benefits of CBD, but few have been proven with reproducible evidence.

Is vaping with marijuana oil or THC oil safer than standard vaping oils? What about vaping devices with essential oils and vitamin mixtures?

There is no form of vaping that is safe. Oil does not belong inside the lungs. All vaping formats have multiple risks of damage to the body and brain. Vitamins are meant to be ingested by mouth or skin and absorbed into the bloodstream. Burning vitamins in liquid form to inhale them has no proven benefit, but the risk of lung damage has already been established. Essential oils may be calming and beneficial when casually inhaled through a diffuser located on the other side of the room. On the other hand, inhaling the oil particles in aerosol format directly into your lungs is a dangerous proposition. The base components of vaping oils are hazardous and potentially cancerous, and no potential benefits from any added elements can outweigh those risks.

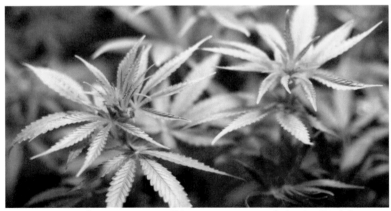

Marijuana plants grow well in many parts of the United States where the weather is warm and favorable for farming. They typically germinate in late spring and are ready for harvest in the late summer to early fall.

The addition of marijuana or THC oil makes a dangerous habit a potentially deadly one. As of February 26, 2020, over 2800 cases of e-cigarette or vaping-associated lung injury (EVALI) requiring hospitalization have been reported in the US, with 60 fatalities confirmed by the CDC. Reporting of these cases abruptly stopped when the COVID-19 pandemic emerged. Despite that, current data suggests a strong association between these hospitalizations and e-cigarette liquids containing tetrahydrocannabinol (THC), vitamin E, or both. A 2020 study of lung fluid from over 50 EVALI patients identified vitamin E, plant oils such as coconut oil, triglyceride oil, and petroleum particles. Non-hospitalized cases of EVALI are not being reported, but we do know the number of individuals experiencing respiratory illness that do not require a hospital stay is greater than the number of cases that do require hospitalization.

A recent case series published in the American Journal of Medicine described the lung damage seen on CT (Computed Tomography) scans of five patients who were hospitalized under the care of physicians at Albany Medical College[x]. All five patients presented with complaints of shortness of breath and fatigue. They admitted to vaping some form of cannabinoid oil in the previous three to six months. CT scans of the chest in all five patients revealed diffuse bilateral ground-glass opacities that spared portions of the extreme periphery of the lungs. The ground-glass pattern terminology is used when lung tissue appears hazy from damage, but not solid like in pneumonia. These findings are different from the lung damage typically seen with traditional non-cannabinoid vaping.

Additionally, the concentration of THC in vaping oils is often much higher than in rolled marijuana joints. In the past, traditional marijuana smoking would not often lead to THC overdose. Because of the low concentration of THC in natural marijuana, the time required to consume an overdose would take hours or more.

Is the additive Vitamin E acetate related to the danger of vaping? Isn't Vitamin E a good thing?

It is true that Vitamin E, also known as alpha-tocopherol, is an important antioxidant that protects the body from damage. Vitamin E is also useful for human development of healthy skin and eyes. However, inhaling vitamin E acetate (VEA) in smoke form does not provide the same effects as eating foods rich in vitamin E or using a vitamin E cream on your skin.

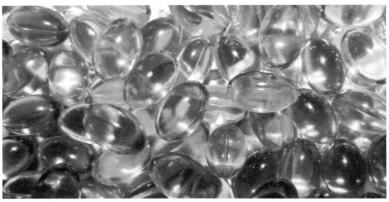

A collection of Vitamin E gel capsules, the safe way to put vitamin E in your body.

Black market THC e-liquid is often watered down from a pure product into diluted forms by cutting the THC oil with vitamin E acetate. This allows the sellers to make more profit from the same amount of raw THC oil. Thousands of e-cigarette smokers and vape pen users have developed respiratory, gastrointestinal, and other bodily symptoms after vaping[xi]. Testing of several samples of underground-economy e-liquids revealed vitamin E acetate within them. A study of 51 patients with e-cigarette or vaping associated lung injury found that 48 of 51 also had deposits of vitamin E acetate in the damaged lung tissue[xii].

Chemical studies have shown that the vitamin E acetate used to dilute THC oil converts to a highly toxic gas when heated to the typical temperatures found in e-cigarettes[xiii]. When tested in animals, VEA inhaled through e-cigarette aerosols caused acute lung injury in the test subjects[xiv].

The vape smoke smells so good, so how can it be bad?

The fruity or candy-inspired scents in vaping smoke come from chemicals added to the vape liquid cartridge. Most of these additives are safe to eat but are not safe to inhale. Imagine if you sprayed air freshener or Lysol spray into a plastic bag. It might smell nice, but you wouldn't want to stick your head into the bag and breathe right out of it. You already know that those chemicals are not safe for you to breathe in directly, but that's very close to what's happening when a person vapes. Dangerous chemicals are released as tiny particles in the vape smoke and those chemicals are inhaled which can damage the lungs.

Chemicals such as diacetyl and 2,3-pentanedione produce a sweet and buttery aroma and are found in dozens of flavor varieties of vape juice[xv]. These chemicals are also linked to patients developing bronchiolitis obliterans[xvi], a severe respiratory disease where chemical particles cause inflammation damage to the smallest airways of the lungs. These tiny branches of our lung system are designed to exchange oxygen and carbon dioxide, but inhaled chemicals damage these passageways causing scarring that blocks the exchange of oxygen and carbon dioxide that is vital for healthy breathing.

These same chemicals were shown to increase risk of lung disease and reduced lung function in the workers exposed to flavoring chemicals of several popcorn production plants[xvii]. A study of urine samples from over a hundred adolescent e-cigarette users revealed significant levels of toxic chemicals in the urine such as acrolein, propylene oxide, and acrylamide.[xviii] Acrolein is a potent pulmonary irritant and carcinogen[xix], which means that breathing in acrolein over a long time could cause lung cancer. Propylene oxide is also a known carcinogen, a chemical that increases your risk of developing cancer.[xx]

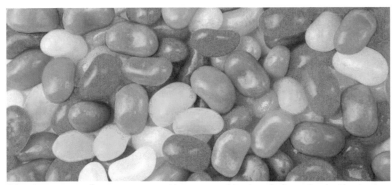

Vaping manufacturers use the same kinds of chemicals that give jellybeans sweet scents to make vaping e-liquid smell desirable. The chemicals are safe to eat, but they are not safe to inhale.

Why are some people dying from this, while many others are doing just fine?

One of the scariest truths regarding the teen vaping epidemic is the fact that one cannot reliably predict the contents of an illegally obtained vape device. Black market salespeople realize that they do not have to maintain customer safety and satisfaction regarding the quality of their product. There's no safety inspection or warning label on the packages to help protect the users. If ingredients are listed, they are usually misleading. A 3% nicotine description on a vape pen might suggest that a low amount of nicotine is being used, but a 3% nicotine concentration in vape juice represents 30 mg/mL concentration, one of the highest concentrations available on the market today. The little transparency that exists cannot be trusted at face value, and the mystery woven into the product only increases the risks to the users.

Although researchers are working hard to find out what is causing healthy people to suddenly die after vaping, there isn't information about why exactly some people suffer serious complications while most others have mild or no symptoms when vaping. This means that we cannot predict what type of people have higher risk of dying or what types of behaviors increase chances of survival. You can search online to find video interviews and news stories of teens having lung failure and even requiring lung transplants to show your children that the negative effects of vaping are serious and unpredictable for users.

Some cases of lung failure have occurred when the chemicals in the e-cigarette aerosolized particles have irritated or injured the inner lining of the lung tissue. This damage results in fluid buildup in the small airways of the lung, which prevents people from breathing normally. Shortness of breath and cough are some early symptoms. Severe damage can lead to hospitalization for lung failure that may require critical care support with a ventilator, and even lead to death.

A recent University of California in San Francisco study of e-cigarette smokers and traditional cigarette smokers found that each group of smokers had elevated levels of biomarkers, which are inflammation-related substances made by the human body, which predicted increased cardiovascular risks[xxi]. Both groups also measured lower flow-mediated dilation than nonusers, meaning blood vessels did not dilate normally in response to increased blood flow within the vessels.

The study also demonstrated that blood vessel damage in smokers is likely caused by airway irritation and inflammation from inhaling chemical irritants. Although each of the common airway irritants was isolated and removed, the presence of any one of the irritants (nicotine, menthol, acrolein, acetaldehyde, or carbon nanoparticles) still led to blood vessel damage after exposure to smoke or aerosols. Another UCSF study exposed rats to cigarette smoke and e-cigarette aerosol and found both groups showed significant increase in blood pressure, decrease in systolic function, and higher susceptibility to developing abnormal heart rhythms like atrial fibrillation and ventricular tachycardia[xxii].

Chapter 2

VAPING DEVICES HIDDEN IN PLAIN SIGHT

The truth might be hiding right under your nose … if only you could see (or smell) it, you might be able to do something about it.

Many parents meticulously childproof their house when their child is a baby or a toddler. However, as they start to grow up, some parents let their guards down. We hope that our children become wiser as they grow older, but as children become teens, they also become more prone to risky behaviors. This chapter provides information about behavior that teens might hide from their parents, so that you are better equipped to identify if your child is hiding risky behavior. We hope to empower parents with the knowledge and confidence to prevent youth substance abuse and to encourage parents to be more curious, vigilant, and involved in their children's lives.

Have you ever wondered what to look for in a child's bedroom and what to say if you find something? Picture a bedroom… a bed, a desk, a chair, a nightstand, posters on the wall, a backpack, and some dirty clothes on the floor. Sounds like a typical tweens or teens' bedroom, right? What if you were putting away clean clothes or looking for a lost library book, and you stumbled across an umbrella that felt too light and opened it to find a flask? Or an

25

unused power strip with a hidden compartment? Parents are often amazed at the items that can easily be hidden from them and the creative devices used to hide them. What shocks them the most is if they imagine that their child may be in possession of a normal-looking item that may be used covertly for drugs or alcohol. It might all be hidden in plain sight. This chapter is an opportunity to explore a teen's bedroom to explain warning signs, coded language, and various trends of youth that may signal drug use, in our efforts to provide guidance on how to have a conversation with youth about substance use.

How do I recognize hidden vaping devices that might be in my home?

As a parent, you may want to investigate a bit more deeply to reassure yourself that your child is not vaping. You may have thought that all vaping devices are shaped like cigars or pens or cigarette-like shapes, but that is far from the truth. Manufacturers of these products now camouflage vaping devices in the form of fake USB flash drives, fake smartwatches, fake pencil sharpeners, and even keychain toys. The possibilities are endless, but here are as many real-world examples as we could find to help you recognize a hidden vaping device in your child's possession.

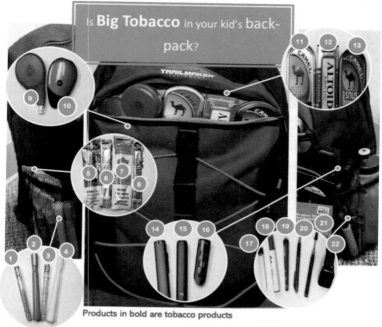

Is **Big Tobacco** in your kid's backpack?

Products in bold are tobacco products

1) **Doob tube**
2) Highlighter
3) **Doob tube**
4) Highlighter
5) **Watermelon Cigarillo**
6) Fruit roll-up
7) **Strawberry Cigarillo**
8) Fruit roll-up

9) White-out
10) **Sourin Drop e-cigarette**
11) **Camel Snus**
12) Altoids mints
13) **Camel Snus**
14) **Vuse e-cigarette**
15) **Blu e-cigarette**

16) USD flash drive
17) **Juul**
18) Marker
19) **Doob tube**
20) Pen
21) **Vape pen**
22) **Vape Watch**

Tobacco products are designed to look like everyday items like candy and school supplies. Don't let the tobacco industry hook your kids for a lifetime of addiction.

A comprehensive display of the many ways vaping and tobacco products could be hidden among the normal items in your child's backpack. Visit https://fortbendcpc.org/ for more information.

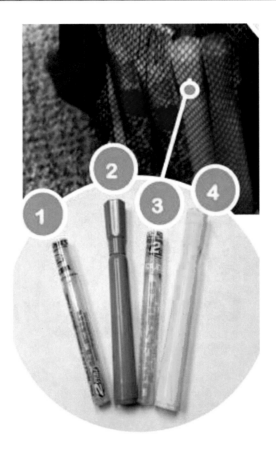

The four objects shown may look like colored pens and highlighters, but items one and three are actually doob tubes, which are small airtight containers that are commonly used to hold cannabis or other marijuana products. Because the doob tube is airtight, teens can hide the strong scent of vaping devices and marijuana products, and camouflage them well enough to carry them to school without parents or teachers noticing.

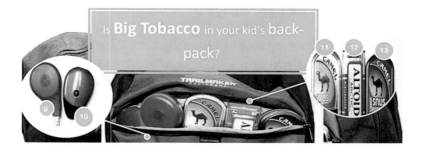

In the picture above, you can see five objects that look like they may belong in a teenager's backpack. Upon closer inspection, some of the items are nicotine products. The two items on the left portion of the open backpack pouch look similar to each other. Item #9 is a white-out correction tool, but item #10 is a Sourin Drop brand e-cigarette device. The three items on the right side of the open pouch are all metal tins that appear to be mints at first glance, but only the middle tin contains a safe food product. Both round containers are tobacco products.

Should I feel ashamed about looking in my child's belongings?

A problem that remains hidden cannot be solved until it's brought out from hiding. If a child is suffering in silence, the sooner you realize it, the sooner you can intervene and help. If you have doubts about what needs to be done, ask yourself what might happen if you sense that something isn't quite right, and you do nothing. Ultimately, the final decision to investigate is yours, but you can seek the opinions of other parents in your social circles, or teachers and counselors at your child's school to get more insight from other adults who interact with your child.

29

How often should I be looking for anything strange?

As a parent, you may want to investigate a bit more deeply or more often if you perceive a significant change in your child's behavior. Trust your child, but also verify that all is well. As you look more closely, take note if you find any of the following:

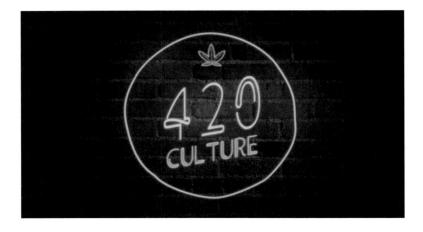

Pro marijuana apparel and posters: 420, 4:20, and 4/20, terms such as "Baked" the color schema of red, yellow, and green have become cultural slang synonymous with themes of marijuana and hashish consumption. April 20th is widely considered "National Marijuana Day," which, for many, is a "counterculture" holiday associated with the celebration and consumption of cannabis use. People who wear apparel or display posters or use anything 420-branded may either have permissive attitudes towards marijuana use or are comfortable with being perceived as a marijuana or cannabis user.

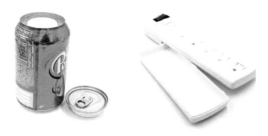

Custom cans and containers with hidden compartments (stash): There are many products available at tobacco/vaping stores and online that appear to be inconspicuous, normal household items but contain hidden compartments. These products are often marketed as diversion safes for storing valuables by hiding them in plain sight, however many teens use them to store drugs.

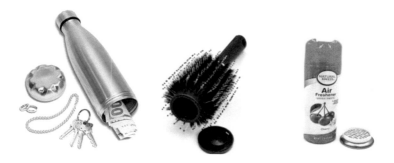

These concealment products come in several forms, including soda cans, energy drinks, water bottles, deodorant, thermos mugs, cleaning products such as kitchen powder cleansers like Ajax or Comet, shaving cream cans, car keys, lipstick/balms, fake plants, candles, clocks, sunglasses, phone cases, and even fake surge protectors. The concealment cans are sometimes weighted to seem as if they contain the actual products they are fashioned after, however it usually doesn't contain anything other than a hollowed-out space to hide drugs and paraphernalia.

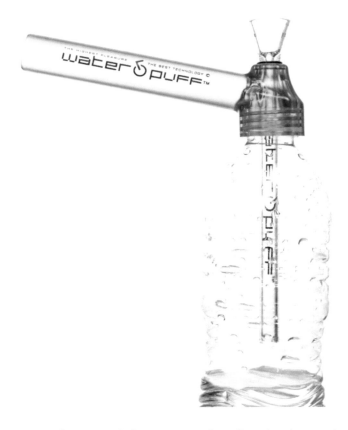

Water Bottle Bong: It is a water pipe disguised as a simple water bottle. It features a screw-on lid that contains the bong (a filtration device) inside the bottle and conceals a hidden ceramic bowl piece below the mouthpiece. Water bongs are used to inhale cannabis, tobacco, or other herbal substances.

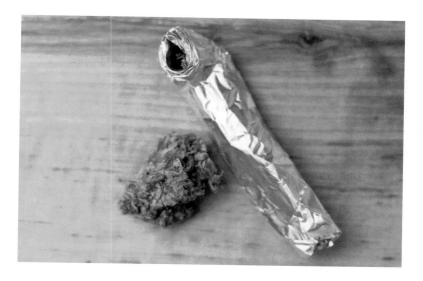

Homemade smoking pipes: Pipes for smoking marijuana can be fashioned out of aluminum foil, soda cans, and water bottles. Even candy and fruit can be used to make pipes. Tutorials on how to make homemade pipes are often available on social media.

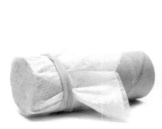 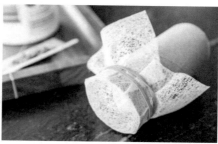

Sploof: a sploof is cylindrical device (typically homemade) that is used as a filtration system to reduce the presence of odor and exhaled smoke after smoking recreational drugs. The device can be made from dryer sheets and a cylindrical object, such as an empty toilet paper roll.

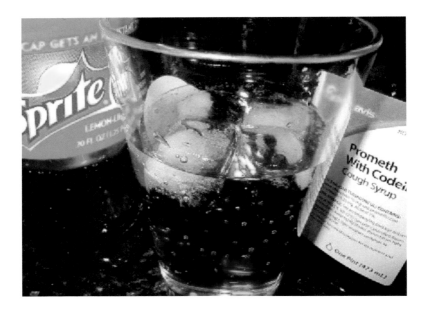

Rx cold medicine, sprite, candy, and **double cup**: Lean, also known as Purple Drank, Syrup, Sizzurp, Dirty Sprite, etc., consists of a mixture of prescription strength cough syrup, containing codeine (an opioid) and promethazine (an antihistamine), soda or other carbonated beverage, and hard candy, such as jolly ranchers. Users are often seen drinking the mixture from two stacked Styrofoam cups. This is because the mixture commonly seeps through the pores of the initial Styrofoam cup, thus users will add a second cup to prevent the residue from seeping through to the outside of the first cup.

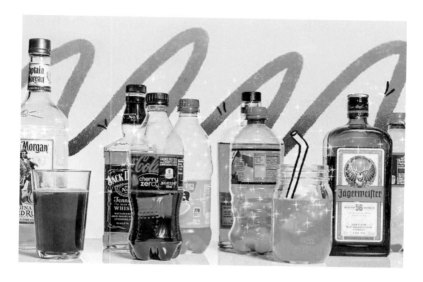

Sports drinks and soda bottles: Sports drinks and soda bottles can easily be used as flasks to conceal alcohol. It can be difficult to detect alcohol when mixed with colored or carbonated liquids. You may have to smell the liquid or even taste it to find out if alcohol is inside.

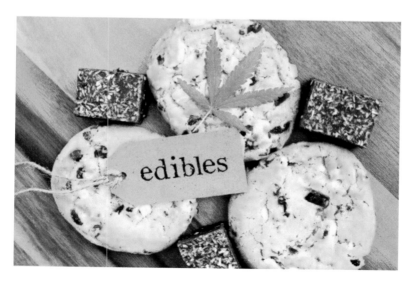

Edibles: Marijuana edibles are food items infused with marijuana/THC. Marijuana edibles have increasingly become more and more popular among young people. The THC takes longer for your body to absorb thus the effects last longer than when it is smoked or vaped. Edibles can last up to 12-24 hrs. Edibles can come in the form of almost any food item, such as cereal bars, pasta, drinks, muffins, coffee, chips, candy, alcohol, etc. Over-consumption is more common with edibles because it can take longer to feel its full effect.

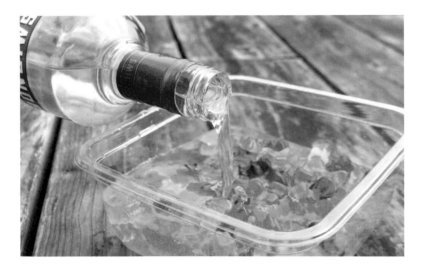

Alcohol-soaked gummy bears: Gummy bears can be soaked in alcohol and camouflaged very easily to appear as normal candy. However, the alcohol-soaked candy will appear slightly bigger if compared side-by-side.

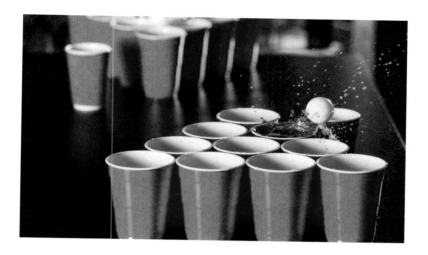

Drinking games: The presence of red solo cups, shot cups or glasses, lots of pennies, or ping pong balls without a paddle can be an indication that young people are playing drinking games, such as beer pong, pennies, or cup stack.

Beer pong is a very popular drinking game, especially among college students, in which two opposing sides throw a table tennis ball into their opponents' cup with the intention of compelling them to drink the contents of the cup in which the ball lands. You probably never played, but you should be able to recognize the components of the game if you see them. Cup stack uses the same materials with different rules.

Pennies is another simple game where players take turns trying to bounce a penny off the table into a short glass. If a player misses, he or she will pass the coin to the next person. The player who gets the penny into the glass then gets to nominate someone to take a drink. Although the name is pennies, the game can be played with any coins.

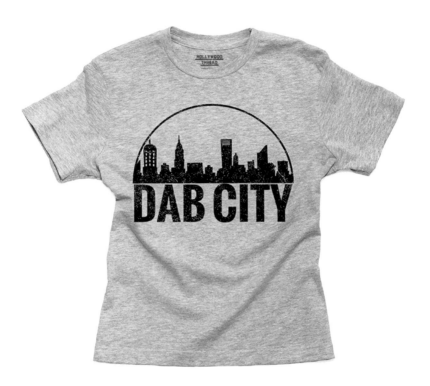

"Dab City" apparel: In the urban dictionary, the term "Dab City" is defined as "a state of consciousness your mind enters after partaking in too many consecutive dabs." "Dab" or "Dabs" are slang for small concentrates of butane hash oil. Hash oil is a wax-like substance containing highly concentrated levels of THC (Tetrahydrocannabinol) extracted from cannabis. Hash oil is extremely potent and can contain 70-90% THC level, competing with the average level of THC in other cannabis products that is about 12%. Users typically utilize vaping devices to ingest a "dab" of the concentrated hash oil. Users call this "dabbing."

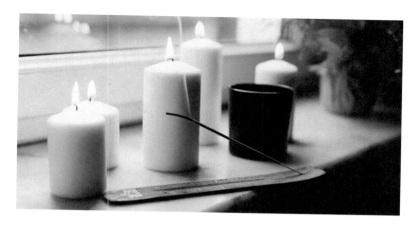

Incense: Incense often has a powerful earthy or floral scent that can be used to cover the smell of marijuana or flavored e-liquid. Frequent use of traditional incense sticks, candles, oil diffusers, and other air sanitizers are commonly used by teens hiding smoking habits.

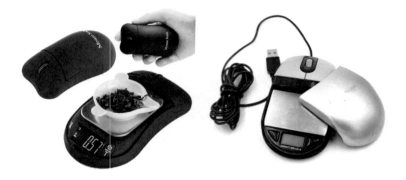

Mouse with a hidden digital scale: Digital scales are more often used to weigh drugs for packaging and distribution than for drug consumption. The mouse functions as both a computer mouse and a concealed digital scale.

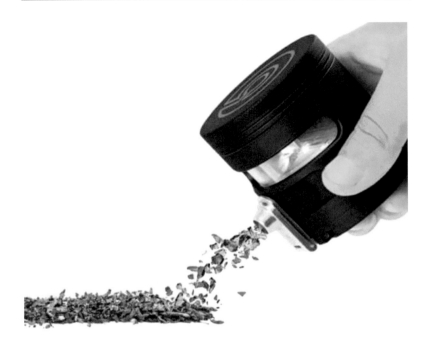

Grinders: A grinder is a tool used to break cannabis buds down into smaller pieces, making it easier to roll into a joint or blunt.

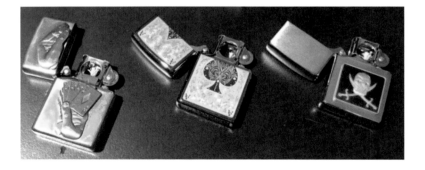

Lighter: The consistent presence of a lighter among an individual's belongings may indicate a habit of smoking marijuana or tobacco products.

40

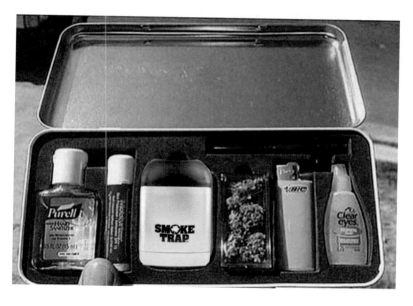

Smoker's kit: A smoker's kit is a collection of items to better hide chronic or habitual use. A regular user or someone who has been frequently caught may purchase or piece together the components of a smoker's kit to continue to use more discreetly. Kits commonly contain a number of concealing items, such as eyedrops to reduce the symptom of eye redness which smokers experience, perfume to conceal smoky odors that normally would attach to clothing and hair, chewing gum or breath mints to conceal smells from the mouth, and hand sanitizer to mask the smell on their fingertips.

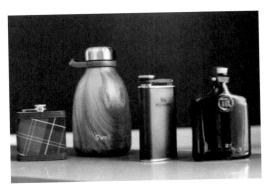
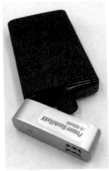

Flasks: Online flasks come in many different shapes and sizes and can be designed to look like household items. We have also seen flip flops with little flasks that fit into the bottom of the shoe, lotion and shampoo bottles that come empty, and sold with a seal to thwart search attempts. There are also flasks shaped like power banks, umbrellas, and tampons, and more deceptive designs all purposely made to conceal the possession of drugs and alcohol.

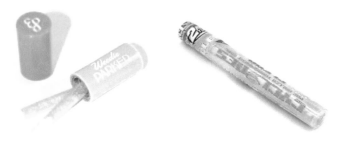

Doob tube: A doob tube is an air-tight container for storing pre-rolled marijuana joints and blunts. These tubes allow users to carry marijuana discreetly. They are typically small and cylindrical and can easily blend in with items in a bag or backpack.

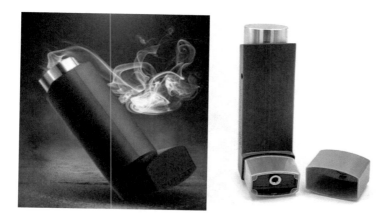

Vape Inhaler: A vaping device designed to look like a medical inhaler. Instead of delivering prescribed drugs, the device functions to aerosolize cannabis, tobacco, or other herbs into microscopic particles that can be inhaled.

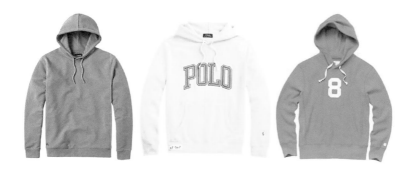

Hoodies: Vape hoodies are a popular way to hide vape pens because normal hoodies are a common item in most teen wardrobes. They are designed to insert a vape pen at the end of one of the hoodie's designed tubed drawstrings and then slide into a discreet pocket, allowing users to inhale through a mouthpiece on the other end of the drawstring.

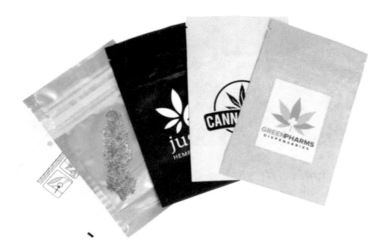

Smell proof bags can be used to conceal the smell of marijuana hidden in a bedroom, a backpack, or during travel in a car or on a school bus.

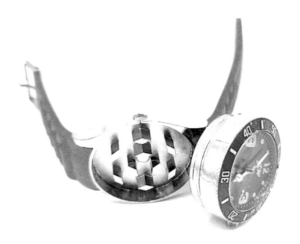

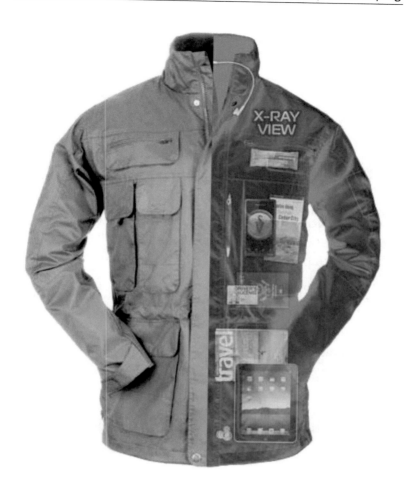

Clothing with hidden pockets: Clothing, such as scarfs, jackets, and shoes with hidden compartments within their lining can be used to hide small flasks, drugs, and paraphernalia. Even watches can hide a secret compartment where drugs can be stashed.

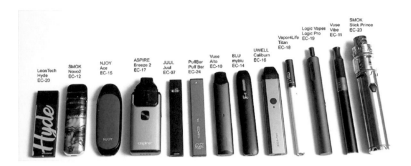

Vaping Devices: Some vaping products are designed to blend into everyday school supplies such as USB-looking e-cigarettes, vape pens (which closely resemble a pen), and smartwatches designed to be used as an e-device. Some of the vaping liquids, e-juice, are flavored to resemble a lot of popular candies.

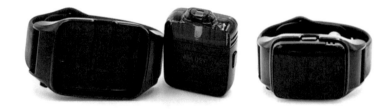

How can I talk to my child about the dangers of vaping?

Talk to your child often to help build an open and trusting relationship. Use everyday opportunities such as sitting at the dinner table or riding in the car to have a lot of little talks rather than focusing on having one big conversation. When you do talk about substance use, express your views with a consistent message. Make sure the information you use during the conversation is age appropriate. Allow your child to ask you questions and pause to listen to their feelings and concerns. Lastly, remember that what you do is just as important as what you say. Our children watch our actions for guidance even more than asking us verbally for instruction.

 **To watch the video walkthrough of our mock bedroom that explains even more detail about vaping devices hidden in plain sight, point your device camera at the QR code!**

Chapter 3

VAPING LAWS AND REGULATIONS

"You have to learn the rules of the game. And then, you have to play better than anyone else."

-Albert Einstein

What is the legal age for vaping?

For nearly three decades in Texas, from 1989 to 2019, the legal age for any tobacco product was 18. In the summer of 2019, the Texas Legislature passed a bill that proposed raising the legal age to purchase tobacco to 21 and the Governor signed it into law shortly afterwards. Marijuana or THC vaping is not and has never been legal in Texas. The Tobacco 21 wave spread to several other states which raised their minimum age to 21 in 2019 also: Arkansas, California, Connecticut, Delaware, Hawaii, Illinois, Maine, Maryland, Massachusetts, New Jersey, New York, Ohio, Oregon, Pennsylvania, Utah, Vermont, Virginia, and Washington. On December 20, 2019, the Federal Food, Drug, and Cosmetic Act was amended to raise the federal minimum age when one can purchase tobacco products to 21 years old.[xxiii] This effectively raises the age to 21 for all states, but each state may have different ways of enforcing this new federal law. Be aware that online retailers may not enforce the new federal law either.

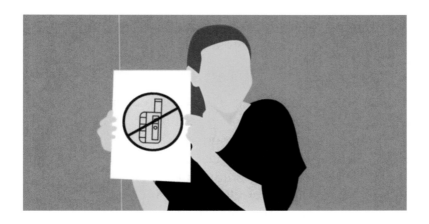

Why hasn't the US Food and Drug Administration (FDA) or local government agencies done more to regulate these products and keep them out of the hands of underage teens?

The FDA claims that it is committed to protecting the public health of all Americans by regulating these addictive products, but it just doesn't feel like they are doing enough. For years, the government politicians promised action on banning flavored vaping liquids, but many of these promises have not been fulfilled. The tobacco companies took quick legal action to block any bans on their products. They also lobbied lawmakers and successfully prevented any further meaningful action to end the sales of flavored e-cigarette liquids. They claim that the sweet and fruity flavors that attract teens to vaping are actually meant for adults to enjoy. This was the same argument Big Tobacco companies made over a decade ago to justify flavored cigarettes. Fortunately for us, in October 2009 the US Congress passed the Family Smoking Prevention and Tobacco Control Act to ban the sale of any cigarette flavors other than menthol and tobacco. Unfortunately, this law did not apply to electronic cigarettes that did not yet exist at the time.

The COVID-19 pandemic has captured much of the attention of the federal government. Prior to the pandemic, our local county sheriffs and police departments engaged in regular monitoring of liquor and vaping stores for selling products to minors. Many of the stores that sell these products closed temporarily during the wave of city shutdowns, but we do not expect to see any change in online purchasing of vaping products. In fact, online purchase and delivery of vaping devices will likely increase to make up for the drop in retail sales. Now more than ever, parents will need to be vigilant in paying attention to the behavior of their teens.

North Carolina became the first state to hold JUUL accountable for its role in the spike of teen vaping abuse after filing a lawsuit in 2019. In June 2021, JUUL agreed to pay a $40 Million settlement to North Carolina for concealing the true risk and danger of the nicotine potency in their products. The lawsuit payments were designated to fund programs to help people quit vaping and prevent e-cigarette addiction.

In April 2022, Juul agreed to a $22.5 million settlement with Washington state to settle lawsuit claims that Juul marketed to minors and lied about the addictive nature of their vaping products. In September 2022, Juul agreed to pay $438 million to settle investigations by over 30 other states regarding how the company marketed to teenagers but did not admit to any wrongdoing.

As of September 30, 2022, all 50 states, Puerto Rico, the District of Columbia, and the US Virgin Islands have all passed laws that prohibit the sale of e-cigarettes to underage persons. After heavy criticism that little was being done to enforce rules around vaping, in October 2022 the FDA asked the DOJ to file injunctions against six companies for the illegal manufacture, sale, and distribution of their e-cigarettes and other vaping products.

In early April 2023, Juul Labs announced a settlement agreement to pay $462 million to six states and the District of Columbia for its role in the teen vaping epidemic. Juul has been repeatedly accused of targeting youth with vibrant ads featuring young people enjoying their products, all while claiming no risks from using their products. The settlement also requires retailers to secure Juul products behind counters and verify the age of the people purchasing them. Juul must also stop using people under the age of 35 in all marketing activities.

Finally, Juul Labs is not the only company being held liable for their actions. Morin Enterprises Inc doing business as E-Cig Crib in Minnesota, Soul Vapor LLC in West Virginia, Super Vape'z LLC in Washington state, Vapor Craft LLC in Georgia, Lucky's Vape & Smoke Shop in Kansas, and Seditious Vapours LLC doing business as Butt Out in the District of Arizona had each been warned by the FDA for marketing, selling, or distributing new tobacco products without FDA preauthorization. The filings would require the companies to permanently stop manufacturing, selling, and distributing their e-cigarettes and other unauthorized vaping products.

Why did the FDA approve vaping if it's not good for you?

The Tobacco Control Act of June 2009 provided the FDA authority to regulate the manufacture, sale, and distribution of tobacco products and devices as well as drugs derived from tobacco. In 2011, a small retrospective survey study showed smokers self-reported significant rates of being able to quit smoking using e-cigarettes, and soon after, the FDA announced that it would regulate e-cigarettes the same way it regulates traditional cigarettes.[xxiv] Any electronic nicotine delivery system (ENDS) on the market after February 15, 2007 was considered a "new" tobacco product that must be authorized by the FDA to be legally sold in the US.

Despite the knowledge of how harmful traditional cigarettes are and how addictive nicotine is, the FDA still allowed the sale of e-cigarettes. In the years that followed, several parties petitioned the FDA to ban or limit e-cigarettes more forcefully, but the electronic cigarette industry and its lobbyists advocated for weaker oversight and even less regulation of their products. Countries around the world began to ban e-cigarettes, while efforts to restrict e-cigarettes in the US remained stagnant.

Since August 2016, the FDA had declined to enforce any premarket authorization requirements on any e-cigarette products. This means that all vaping products were under the authority of the FDA but marketed to the public in an unauthorized status. These companies were not worried about punishment because the FDA has not chosen to enforce the law against any company selling these products. In 2019, the FDA issued warning letters to six companies advising them to remove a total of 71 products from the market.

As of October 2019, the US Food and Drug Administration strengthened its warning to the public to stop the use and avoid starting use of vaping products that contain tetrahydrocannabinol (THC), the psychoactive component of marijuana. The FDA also advises against use of any vaping product purchased on "the street," online, or on social media, which would include all methods by which teenagers currently obtain vaping products. The FDA has also worked with eBay to remove JUUL listings and prevent new listings for ENDS. The FDA has also sent dozens of warning letters to companies who appear to market e-liquids with misleading labeling that appeal to children or use social media influencers in violation of FDA guidelines.

Prior to 2020, there was no pre-approval process for these products, which means that no pre-market testing by FDA was conducted, and no current products are pre-approved for use prior to being sold to the public. The FDA set a deadline in September 2020 for companies to file applications to seek permission from the FDA to continue selling vaping products.

Unfortunately, in October of 2021, the FDA authorized the marketing and sale of electronic nicotine delivery systems for the first time in its history. The company Vuse applied for approval for its tobacco-flavored e-liquid products. Although ten other fruity-flavored products were denied, the approval of new e-cigarettes was a step backwards towards our mission to end teen vaping. As of January

2023, the FDA reports that it has not approved any vaping product for use in quitting smoking or any other health benefit. No ENDS has been approved by the FDA to market any claim of reduced risk or harm reduction in comparison to traditional cigarettes. All products on the market today are approved for recreational use in adults only.

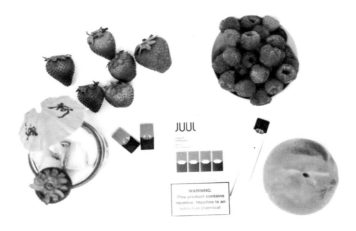

A Juul advertisement highlighting some of their most popular fruity flavor nicotine offerings: pina colada, strawberry, raspberry, and peach.

Why are they allowed to sell in kid-appealing fruity flavors?

In 2015, the FDA drew up plans for a ban on all flavored vaping liquids, but dozens of lobbyists persuaded the government not to move forward with the flavor ban. In 2018, Juul stopped selling some of their flavored products in stores under heavy pressure from the FDA. Flavored tobacco products were generating between $10 million and $100 million each month for Juul. Although Juul pulled many sweet smell nicotine pods from the market, other companies continued to sell them, and they were often compatible with Juul devices.

In June 2019, San Francisco was the first major US city to ban fruit and sweet flavored vaping (actually, they banned all vaping products). In September of 2019, Michigan became the first state to ban sweet and fruit flavored e-cigarette liquid with a six-month ban that required renewal every six months. New York's Governor issued a similar ban by executive order, but it was blocked by a lawsuit and is not currently in effect. Also, in September of 2019, Massachusetts legislators passed a ban on all vape sales, both marijuana and tobacco e-cigarettes of any kind, but the ban only lasted four months. Rhode Island's Governor implemented a similar four-month ban on flavored electronic cigarettes that has the option to be extended as well.

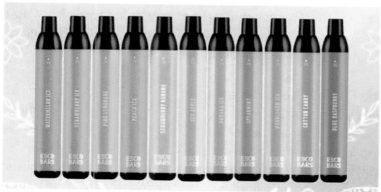

Here's a colorful collection of flavored disposable vaping devices called Escobars. They are not FDA approved, but they are widely available in the US.

In October 2019, Washington state enacted an emergency rule banning flavored vaping products for four months. Oregon legislators enacted a six-month statewide ban on flavored nicotine and marijuana e-cigarette products except for products that contain 100% pure marijuana terpenes. Montana also implemented a four-month ban on all flavored nicotine, THC, and CBD vaping products.

On January 2, 2020, the FDA released a policy update that calls for companies to cease manufacturing, distribution, and selling of any flavor cartridge-based e-cigarettes (except menthol). Unfortunately, this policy update is not a complete ban on sweet-flavored vape juice. Companies can apply for FDA approval for all flavors, and some have already applied. Any company that submits a product application will be allowed to sell any of their flavored products for an additional year, as allowed by individual state and local regulations. The policy also permits flavored nicotine in disposable devices that cannot be refilled This means that teens may shift away from Juul and refillable vape mods and use disposable flavored e-cigarettes like Puff Bars instead.

The FDA has been delaying the full implementation of this policy for months, but a court order set a firm deadline. The court order gives the FDA a year to review all applications and determine which products are safe for continued sale. This means that teens will still be tempted by flavored vaping liquids for many months to come.

Is vaping prohibited for students on the campus of Texas public schools?

Yes, the Texas Education Code is state law that prohibits students from smoking, using, or possessing e-cigarettes and all other electronic vaporizing devices at school. It also extends the prohibition to any school-related or school-sanctioned activities whether they are on or off school property[xxv].

Is vaping allowed for adults on school property or at school-related events?

No, the Texas Education Code also prohibits adults from smoking, using, or possessing e-cigarettes and all other tobacco products at any school or school-sanctioned activity, both on-campus and off school property. This prohibition covers all individuals, whether they are teachers, other employees, adult students, parents, volunteers, or visitors.

Why would they sell vaping devices that could kill you?

Our government does not make products illegal simply because the product may cause death. Despite the large number of people who die from diseases related to alcohol or tobacco products, both tobacco and alcohol are available for sale at every corner. The sad truth is that the government will allow dangerous products to be sold if they can have a share in the profits of those sales. The government warns the public about risky consumer products but allows each person to decide what to consume and what not to consume. Although most products that have little or no benefit, such as cocaine or nicotine, are tightly restricted, the US government continues to allow widespread sale of nicotine products.

In 2016, the Child Nicotine Poisoning Prevention Act required packaging for e-liquid containers to meet current standards for all other products for prevention of child poisoning. The US Department of Transportation banned use of e-cigarettes on airplanes[xxvi], but no other bans from the government have been enacted. In November 2016, the US Department of Housing formally banned cigarette smoking in public housing and purposefully declined to ban e-cigarettes.[xxvii]

The Preventing Online Sales of E-Cigarettes to Children Act (known also as "the Vape Mail Ban") was passed as part of the fiscal year 2021 omnibus spending bill, US HR133. One section of the bill amends the PACT Act to include vaping products in its list of products prohibited from delivery by mail. As of September 9, 2021, any e-cigarette or vaping product not specifically authorized by the FDA is illegal. Most companies selling products nationwide have permission from the FDA to sell to adults. To date, no e-cigarette or vaping device has been approved as a cessation device or authorized to make any claims that vaping is less harmful than traditional cigarettes.

In late June 2022, the FDA ordered Juul Labs Inc. to remove all its e-cigarettes from the U.S. market, after increased scrutiny related to its marketing to teens. Soon after, a U.S. court of appeals granted Juul an emergency stay, temporarily blocking the FDA's order. Then, in early July, the FDA temporarily paused its order to investigate the company's application for FDA permission to sell its products again. Unfortunately, when it seems like the country is taking a step forward to control underage vaping, we take one or two steps backwards as well.

Do other countries ban vaping products?

Beginning over ten years ago, several countries partially or completely banned e-cigarettes and vaping products. Most countries have no laws prohibiting people from vaping, but the sale of vaping products is illegal, such as in Antigua and Barbuda, Argentina, Brazil, Colombia, Chile, Egypt, Hong Kong, India, Panama, Saudi Arabia, Sri Lanka, and Thailand all have robust bans on the sale of e-cigarettes and vaping products. Other countries like Mexico, Nicaragua, North Korea, Qatar, Singapore, and Cambodia ban all vaping devices and electronic cigarettes. Australia bans all nicotine e-cigarettes unless prescribed by a medical professional.

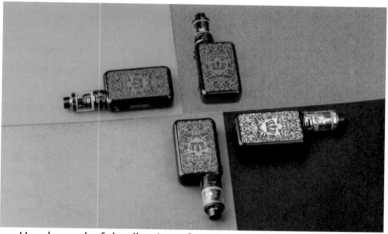

Here's a colorful collection of vaping devices that are small enough to conceal in the palm of your hand. It's hard to imagine that the bright colors and sweet flavors were not intentionally aimed at younger users.

Chapter 4

THE REAL TRUTH ABOUT TEEN VAPING

There's an old saying – what you don't know can't hurt you. That saying is completely wrong. Knowledge is power in the fight to save your teens. Going into battle ignorant of the truth is the same as entering the fight unarmed. Here's the highlights of what the e-cigarette companies don't want you to know.

How common is teen vaping?

The 2022 National Youth Tobacco Survey (NYTS) results on e-cigarettes use showed that over three million middle and high school students reported current use of e-cigarettes of some kind within the past 30 days. Separated by age group, 1 in 6 high school students is vaping and 1 in 20 middle school students is vaping. The NYTS is conducted every year by the FDA and Centers for Disease Control and Prevention (CDC)[ii]. The results of the 2022 NYTS survey represent an increase in the number of teens vaping when compared to the results of the 2021 NYTS survey.

Why is vaping so attractive to teens?

Advertising campaigns have portrayed vaping as a safe recreational activity by using famous actors and actresses and social media influencers to normalize the activity. Movie scenes and social media live streams are advertising for vaping while parents may not even recognize it. Social media influencers have millions of teenage followers emulating their behavior. Vaping companies can pay influencers to use their products during normal daily life. Vaping has become a social activity among teens, and they congregate to vape like how adults meet up to have coffee. Teenagers are also engaging in smoke tricks just like people did with traditional cigarettes in the past, but these vape smoke performances now reach a much larger audience through social media. Search "vape tricks" online and you should see dozens of videos showing smoking tricks on YouTube and other video websites. Teens think these tricks are cool and they emulate them and then show them to their friends both in person and online.

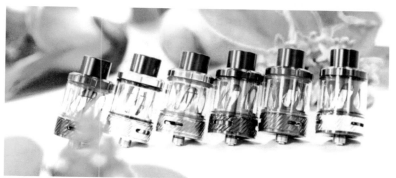

An ad image of vaping devices that look more like toys than dangerous drug delivery systems they are.

If vaping is illegal for kids, how are they getting the vaping devices into schools?

Teenagers have a variety of methods of circumventing the

legal restrictions to obtain vaping devices and e-liquid. As with alcohol and standard cigarettes, teenagers often find adults who are willing to assist in the purchase of these items. Teenagers will also utilize connections with older siblings or older classmates who have become legal adults to access e-cigarettes and vaping devices. The students who gain illegal access will often share that access with other students, sometimes to gain popularity or for financial gain.

With vaping, teenagers can also use social media to browse black market websites and illegal distributors' inventory of vaping options and make purchases on Snapchat or Instagram through their cell phone. After they make payment with apps like the Cash app or Venmo, they can have the purchase delivered to a friend's house or even their own home without their parents' knowledge. Kids can even arrange for delivery in private areas of public spaces like movie theaters and shopping malls. Because the devices are so small, once purchased, teens usually don't have any problems sneaking them into schools.

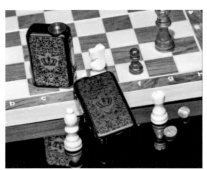 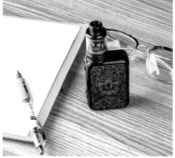

Vaping devices are designed to blend in with everyday items so that youth are conditioned to think that vaping is normal, and adults are conditioned to ignore the devices.

Online marketplaces also give teenagers the option to purchase vaping devices and e-liquid without age verification and with the benefit of home delivery. These teenagers who obtain vaping devices illicitly then take them to school and resell to other students.

Brick and mortar vape shops have also increased in number significantly over the years. While many follow the rule of law, many others do not check the ID of everyone who purchases vaping devices. Gas stations are also notorious for failing to check ID consistently to allow them to sell illegal items to underage minors.

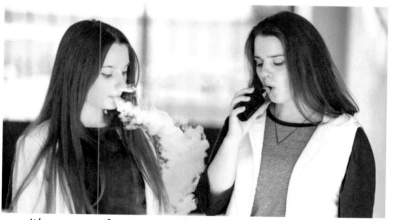

It's common for teens to share a vaping device, which is dangerous on multiple levels.

How can kids afford to vape? Is it an expensive habit?

Several e-cigarette companies offer their products at a significant discount, such as 99 cents, for new customers. This advertising gimmick is used as a lure to try vaping, despite the decades of evidence proving nicotine is addictive and that a significant proportion of first-time users will continue long-term nicotine use. Refill cartridges are not expensive, and black-market cartridges can be even less expensive. Students have been reported selling short-term use of their vape devices for as little as one dollar for a "hit" of vape juice. This means that it would not take much money to start this dangerous habit. Once addicted, it can become an expensive habit to maintain, which seems to be the goal of the corporations behind vaping. They want kids hooked so that they can stay in business for years to come.

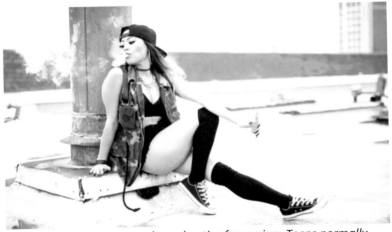

This photo was created to advertise for vaping. Teens normally wouldn't have access to commercial rooftops and modern vaping devices allow teens to vape indoors without being detected.

Why is vaping so addictive?

Vaping is addictive because the nicotine within is a powerfully addictive drug. Nicotine alters your brain chemistry and increases cravings for more nicotine, causing a vicious cycle of reinforcing the addiction. Past

64

research on nicotine in tobacco cigarettes documented higher potential for addiction with faster delivery of nicotine and higher concentration of nicotine. Depending on the type of e-liquid, vaping can deliver nicotine faster and in higher concentrations than standard cigarettes.[xxviii] A single Juul pod may contain as much nicotine as an entire pack of cigarettes.[xxix] Nicotine levels in blood after inhaling reach a peak at about 10 minutes, but nicotine can reach the brain in as little as 10 seconds.[xxx]

Teenagers are especially susceptible to nicotine addiction. In young people, addiction can result from as little as 5mg of nicotine a day, which is about one-fourth of a vape liquid pod. When nicotine reaches the brain, it causes the release of dopamine and several other neurochemicals. Because the adolescent brain matures as the network of dopamine receptors evolves, nicotine disrupts the process as it creates an addictive feedback loop that reinforces even more nicotine use.[xxxi] Long-term nicotine use in adolescents can cause irreversible changes in the brain that may manifest as irritability, increased impulsivity, and mood disorders.

What makes vaping so dangerous?

For decades, studies have shown that nicotine has irreversible effects on the brain. Newer studies establish a link between vaping and both lung damage and increased risk of heart disease. In a recent study, researchers compared blood samples from e-cigarette smokers, traditional cigarette smokers, and non-smokers and the blood from the e-cigarette smokers. The blood vessel cells from both types of smokers showed reduced ability to circulate blood and increased levels of hydrogen peroxide and reduced levels of blood vessel permeability and nitric oxide production, which suggests increased risk of developing cardiovascular disease with prolonged use[xxxii].

We can all agree that teenage brain is not fully matured, but the brain actually does not finish development until age 25 or later[xxxiii]. The section of the brain responsible for planning, prioritizing, and making good decisions, called the prefrontal cortex, is the last to fully mature. It is also no coincidence that auto insurance companies charge much higher premiums for drivers under the age of 25.

When nicotine interacts with a brain before maturity is complete, it can disrupt the formation of brain circuits that control attention and interfere with adolescent development of executive functioning and inhibition control[xxxiv]. Essentially the drug can rewire the young brain to underestimate risk in the future and chase after unhealthy rewards more often.

Is the rise in vaping connected to the fall in cigarette smoking?

Traditional tobacco use has been declining in the US for years, especially in the younger population. Educational campaigns successfully communicated the dangers of smoking cigarettes so well that kids today still perceive cigarettes as a bad thing. It seems that big tobacco companies saw the popularity in e-cigarette use among this generation as a way to modernize their business. After e-cigarettes sales rose significantly in the early 2000s, major tobacco companies began purchasing existing e-cigarette companies or developing their own e-cigarette products. They also figured out that alternative names like vaping would help electronic cigarettes escape the stigma of traditional cigarettes.

Big Tobacco companies were ready to invest big money into vaping. The Altria Group (formerly Philip Morris Companies) purchased a 35% stake in Juul Labs for over $12 billion dollars in 2018. Imperial Brands Tobacco Company fully purchased Blu e-cigarettes from the Reynolds Tobacco Company, while Reynolds created its own brand of e-cigarettes called Vuse. The British American Tobacco company sells Vype. These companies invested heavily in the success of e-cigarettes and seem to be applying their lobbying efforts and advertising methods toward the same goal. These companies advertise on platforms that teenagers prefer, such as Snapchat, Spotify, and Instagram, because they want these young individuals to get hooked on their products.

How are kids able to vape at school without teachers or administrators finding out?

Teenagers today are very resourceful – they observe and adapt to changing circumstances. The act of vaping takes only a second, and the vaping paraphernalia currently available can hide vaping devices in plain sight. Students have reported that they can activate the device and use it in the brief moments a teacher has turned around to write something on the board. They will tell you that classmates will use social media and communication apps to covertly plan how to vape between classes. They convene in different bathrooms at school on a rotating schedule to avoid detection. They even monitor the halls for approaching teachers to prevent each other from getting caught. Because the vape smoke from e-cigarettes dissipates so quickly, teachers may only catch the faint scent of bubble gum or vanilla spice or fruit punch in the air. Teachers may mistake the remnants for body splash or perfume, but even if they do suspect vaping in class, they would not be able to attribute the smell to any one student. Students can also hide the vape smoke by exhaling into their shirt or sleeve. All of these complexities combine to create a situation where it can be very difficult to catch kids vaping in the act.

If my child is caught vaping at school, what might happen? What are the possible penalties?

When a child is caught vaping, the prohibited items are confiscated, and local authorities are notified. Most school districts have strict policies related to tobacco possession and use on campus, giving in-school suspension or warnings with counseling for the first offense. Additional offenses might result in longer suspensions or placement in a Disciplinary Alternative Education Program (DAEP). However, if the e-liquid cartridge tests positive for marijuana in any amount, the offense becomes more serious because marijuana is a controlled substance. This leads to mandatory removal of the child off campus to a DAEP for up to a year.

When marijuana or other controlled substances are involved, expulsion also becomes an option for punishment, with possible placement in the local county equivalent of a Juvenile Justice Alternative Education

Program. The authorities also have the right to charge your child with possession of a controlled substance and weigh the entire e-liquid vial to determine the level of criminal charges, which would make it much more likely that your child may go to jail.

Most states have a low threshold of four ounces for marijuana possession to be considered a misdemeanor. If your child is found to have vape juice weighing above the state weight limit, possession becomes a felony. In Texas, Arkansas, Massachusetts, and Oregon, the limit is 4 oz, but in Nevada, Georgia, South Carolina, Florida, classify felony possession at 1 oz of marijuana. Some states have no felony charges regardless of weight, including California, Iowa, Michigan, and Virginia, while other states classify marijuana possession as a felony with any amount no matter how small, like Arizona, Oklahoma, Kansas, and Wisconsin. Most vape juice vials are heavy enough to trigger a felony violation because the authorities usually weigh the entire vial or cartridge, not just the liquid. Your teen should be aware that a felony conviction is more than just time in jail. Felons lose the right to vote, the right to own a gun, the right to serve as a police officer, and potentially more depending on your state laws. Felons also have a harder time finding work and getting into college.

Is there some kind of drug test to find out if my child is vaping?

Currently, standard urine drug tests can identify marijuana as well as over a dozen different drugs of abuse, but nicotine is not one of them. To test specifically for nicotine use, a specialized drug test is needed, one designed to pick up nicotine, or its common byproduct cotinine. These tests are run in larger labs and most clinics can collect a urine sample from the patient for rapid transport to the lab, but the test is quite expensive, usually over $100. At Quest Diagnostics, the urine test for nicotine and cotinine (test code 90646) needs only 1 mL of urine and can detect cotinine several days after the last nicotine product use and provides results in 3 days.[xxxv] Some instant nicotine tests can be purchased online, but it would be hard to assess the accuracy or reliability of lab tests purchased online. Proper testing at a medical facility would be the safe and prudent approach.

Chapter 5

KEEP IT REAL WITH YOUR KIDS: A HEART-TO-HEART VAPING DISCUSSION

"An ounce of prevention is worth a pound of cure."

-Benjamin Franklin

We've all seen the long-term effects of tobacco and cigarette use and nicotine addiction over the decades. Wouldn't it be nice if we could prevent the next generation from suffering a similar fate? Your children might already have their minds made up about vaping, and if so, they probably know that you won't agree with them. Knowing the signs of vaping use will help you identify those signs better, even when the child is trying to hide it.

How can I tell if my child is vaping?

The signs of nicotine use can be very subtle. Nicotine use can sometimes cause headache, dizziness, agitation, fatigue, restlessness, or confusion. If vape juice is ingested orally, you may notice nausea, vomiting, abdominal burning pain, or diarrhea. Nicotine overdose can cause rapid heart rate and high blood pressure or low heart rate and low blood pressure, respiratory distress (trouble breathing), seizures, and coma.[xxxvi] Because of the short half-life of nicotine, it is possible to experience signs of withdrawal just a few hours after the last use such as anxiety, irritability, anger, or depressed mood.

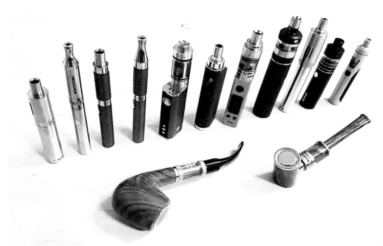

Here's a variety of electronic cigarettes, electronic pipes, and vape pens. The more you see them, the easier it will be to recognize them.

By paying close attention to your child, you may pick up on other behavioral changes of nicotine withdrawal such as increased appetite, restlessness, difficulty falling asleep or trouble staying asleep. If your child tries to quit without help, you may notice more severe signs of nicotine withdrawal.

Teens who vape may develop signs and symptoms of EVALI, such as shortness of breath, cough, chest pain, diarrhea, fever, fatigue, or abdominal pain. These symptoms can occur within hours of use, or after days or weeks of continued e-cigarette use. Because these symptoms are common in many illnesses, it would be difficult for parents to know how to interpret these symptoms, but a lack of improvement with traditional medical treatments should lead parents to consider alternative causes.

As a parent, you may want to investigate a bit more deeply to reassure yourself that your child is not vaping. You may have thought that all vaping devices are shaped like cigars or pens or cigarette-like shapes, but that is far from the truth. Manufacturers of these products now camouflage vaping devices in the form of fake USB flash drives, fake smartwatches, fake pencil sharpeners, and even keychain toys. Consider checking out your child's web browsing history and YouTube viewing history to see if they have been researching vaping. They may consider it an invasion of privacy, but you have the right as a parent to supervise their activities, especially while they live under your roof.

How can I keep my child from starting?

An open dialogue with your child about vaping is a good way to start the process of educating him or her about the risks of vaping. Depending on age, your teen probably already has some information about vaping and some of that will be misconception or falsehoods spread by marketing from the manufacturers. Use educational materials from the reference section at the end of this guide to download activities and flyers that will help your child understand the truth about vaping.

If you worry that using vaping devices or other electronic cigarettes may lead to other drug abuse, your fears are valid. Proponents of e-cigarettes argue that they act as a way for traditional cigarette smokers to transition away from cigarettes to e-cigs to non-smoker status. However, the research evidence linking teen vaping to increased teen cigarette smoking and other drug use is growing.[xxxvii] Vaping has no benefits for teens, only harm at the time they use them and risk of more harm in the future. The research into the long-term effects of vaping is only beginning.

Why is it that my child just can't see how dangerous vaping is? Why would they do something so dangerous?

Unfortunately, most teenagers just don't perceive risk the way adults do. Children sometimes see risk as a challenge, like hang-gliding off the side of a mountain or like a street drag race that needs to be won. Teenagers especially fall victim to the fallacy of thinking "bad things could happen, but not to me" which allows them to justify engaging in dangerous behavior. Even level-headed teens may perceive e-cigarettes as safer than traditional cigarettes and falsely interpret that difference in risk as actual safety.

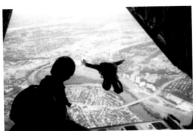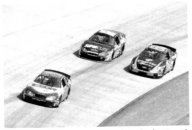

A man skydiving (left). A professional race car event (right). Both activities are considered high-risk, but media and advertising have conditioned people to perceive both activities as interesting and exciting.

Teens seem to accept the fact that traditional cigarette smoking is bad for their health and can lead to lung cancer and death. Because e-cigarettes are so new in comparison, the history of consequences is not as deep, so it is easier to believe marketing that claims vaping is safe. Unfortunately, vaping could lead to lung disease much more quickly than smoking traditional cigarettes, causing disease and death in months instead of decades.

Kids today are bombarded with both overt and subliminal advertising that promotes vaping and other e-cigarette use. In the absence of an equal amount of negative messaging, teems may be swayed to believe that vaping is safe and acceptable.

Teens may also intentionally use vaping like other drugs, as a way to cope with stressful circumstances. I recently counseled a parent whose son began vaping not long after he learned that his parents were divorcing. The child became depressed, and friends offered vaping as a way for him to feel better about his situation. The pandemic created more stress and anxiety in our teens than we may realize. Many studies have surveyed teens and shown that extraordinary pandemic-related life changes were stressful and led to measurable increases in anxiety symptoms and depression symptoms[xxxviii], and even changes in brain structure on MRI scans[xxxix].

My child is already vaping. How do I help my child quit?

If your child is already vaping on a regular basis, your child is probably already addicted to nicotine and will likely have a difficult time quitting, but with help, it can be accomplished. Help is available to anyone by calling 1-800-QUIT-NOW or 1-877-44U-QUIT where counselors will listen to your situation and assist you with developing a game plan. Parents can visit www.smokefree.gov with their teens for a variety of assistance methods to quit. They offer free programs that give advice and encouragement through text messaging 24 hours a day, 7 days a week. They also offer smartphone apps for both Android and Apple phones that provide personalized advice based on individual smoking patterns, quitting goals, and motivations to quit. Smokefree.gov also has active social media profiles and teens can visit them for support and encouragement, or parents can visit the profiles and repost or forward the messages to their teens.

The process of trying to quit vaping or e-smoking feels different for each person, but everyone will experience some variation of nicotine withdrawal symptoms. The nicotine cravings can manifest as a mild urge or an intense desire to vape or smoke. Nicotine substitution medication like gum and patches are helpful, but usually require a prescription. Distracting activities can divert your attention away from the cravings, like playing a sport or a game. Occupying your hands is another helpful tactic, by doodling, typing, or using a squeeze ball stress reliever.

At times, the withdrawal symptoms will feel like restlessness, irritability, or feeling jumpy. If you know that you should expect these feelings, you can help your child prepare both mind and body to deal with them. Go together for a jog or a walk if he or she feels restless. A quick physical activity break can help shake loose from feeling jittery. Remind yourself and your child that their body feels this way because it's getting used to living without nicotine.

Another common symptom of nicotine withdrawal is difficulty falling asleep or trouble staying asleep. If you are using any nicotine replacements, do not use them for at least an hour before bedtime, as nicotine can make it harder for you to fall asleep. Caffeine lasts longer in your body after you stop using nicotine, so remember to avoid coffee, tea, and other caffeinated drinks in the afternoon and evening. Traditional tips like avoiding TV before bedtime and avoiding heavy meals before bed are also helpful with maintaining good sleep habits after your child quits vaping.

As the body adjusts to living without nicotine, it's normal for the appetite to increase. The stress of quitting can trigger nervous eating habits, but staying active can calm down the urges to eat when nervous or bored. When it's time for a snack, choose healthy snack options like nuts and veggies or sugar-free snacks to minimize the effects on your daily calorie intake.

Breaking an addiction requires the efforts of a team, not just individual willpower. Alone, a person fighting to beat nicotine addiction may feel anxious, sad, or depressed at times, but the connections with family and friends who are supportive help fight against those negative emotions. It is important to understand that people who have help are much more successful at quitting than people who try alone. Your support is a very important part of your child's journey to becoming nicotine-free.

What should I do if my child seems to be having a bad reaction to vaping?

If you suspect your child has become ill from vaping or if you know your child is vaping and appears to be having a hard time breathing, you should immediately yell for help. If nearby help is not available, you should call 9-1-1. If your child can stand, help move your child into a fresh air environment. If your child cannot move, do not move your child without the guidance of a professional. Evaluate the child for a heartbeat and breathing. If there is no heartbeat, begin CPR chest compressions. If there is no breathing, provide rescue breathing. Continue these lifesaving measures until paramedics or other qualified help arrives to assist you.

If the situation does not seem like an emergency, you can call your child's Pediatrician for advice or take your child to the nearest Urgent Care Clinic or Minor Emergency Center for a rapid evaluation. Once the situation is under control, be sure to notify the FDA by submitting details of the symptoms and the device through a confidential online Safety Reporting Portal at www.safetyreporting.hhs.gov.

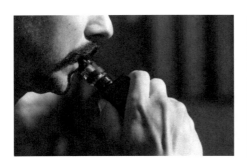
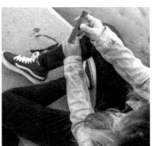

What can we do to raise awareness of this public safety hazard?

The FDA has partnered with Scholastic to develop educational materials to post in schools and display to kids. You can download the posters for free at http://www.scholastic.com/youthvapingrisks/ and share them with your child's teacher and engage with the school's nurse and counselors to raise awareness at school. You can work with your community leaders to host a local event like a Town Hall where local experts can answer questions from the community. You can also share this information with your community groups or church groups to get the word out to other parents.

My teens are 18 and 19 and they don't take the dangers of vaping seriously. How do I convince them that they shouldn't vape now or ever?

We've always known that there are no proven benefits of vaping for non-smokers. This is not an issue under debate. Vaping does no good. It provides no health benefits. When traditional cigarettes were first introduced, they were believed to be good for promoting weight loss. Many years later, the real danger of lung destruction and lung cancer became clear. Fortunately, we did not have to wait decades to learn that vaping is harmful. We have that knowledge now and we must share these truths to fight against the misleading marketing designed to get people addicted to nicotine.

How can I help my teen prepare for the peer pressure environment that will likely lead to a friend offering a vaping device to my child?

Teen vaping is so commonplace, it is almost certain that your child will find himself or herself in a situation where others are vaping. The time will come when a friend asks your child, "Do you want to try some?" Time will slow to a crawl as the eyes of their classmates stare, waiting for a response. Your child may know the risks of vaping, but also fear that saying no could lead to social ridicule. This internal struggle happens every day, and not every child makes the right choice.

The pressure to say yes is real, but you can help your child be ready for this inevitable moment. By role-playing with your teen, you can prepare for these tense moments. Your child should have a variety of responses ready to defend them from peer pressure. Whether it's a genuine concern for sharing a mouthpiece and spreading germs or a threat of asthma returning from early childhood, you can come up with a few ways to say no and not suffer the social consequences of looking like an outcast.

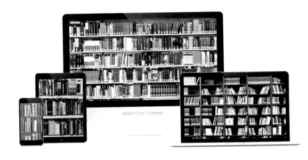

Do our children receive any in-school education programs to educate them about e-cigarettes and vaping?

Most middle and high schools teach a semester of health education as part of the PE curriculum. During this course, the teachers usually present a module on drug abuse prevention. These modules are broad and may or may not cover vaping dangers. Printed textbooks may be outdated and may not have any up-to-date information on the risks of vaping. Some school districts are integrating online education into these health classes, using interactive websites like CATCH My Breath – An online nicotine vaping prevention program, available at the website https://www.catch.org/bundles/23725 and ASPIRE: A Smoking Prevention Interactive Experience. www.aspire2.mdanderson.org.

CATCH My Breath is the only evidence-based youth nicotine vaping prevention program for grades 5-12 that has been proven to significantly reduce student's chances of vaping. It includes grade-level specific education with a variety of supplemental materials, self-paced modules, and virtual field trips. CATCH Global Foundation also provides training for teachers and health educators to help ensure effective delivery of the vape education program. We suggest that you reach out to your school administrators to discuss the details of the health education components and respectfully request that vaping education be included in the curriculum. The more kids we educate on the risks of vaping, the more likely those kids are to become victims to the vaping epidemic.

Each school district has a local health advisory council that is required by law to publish a notice in the student handbook and on the district's website that the district maintains and enforces policies that prescribe penalties for tobacco product and e-cigarette use. The school health advisory councils are also tasked with recommending instruction to prevent substance abuse, but that does not always mean students learn specifically about vaping risks.

What else can we do to get our government to better protect our kids from this danger?

Several government agencies are working hard to combat the teen vaping epidemic. Use of nicotine and THC in all forms is already prohibited for all children in nearly every state. To better protect our children, we need to contact our government representatives in local, state, and federal government to let them know that we take this epidemic seriously. If the people who claim to represent us do not fight to protect us, we must look to elect new representatives who will work towards our best interests.

We must speak with one voice and demand a ban on flavored vaping liquid and that the ban be enforced seriously. We need to request tighter regulations on imports to prevent illicit distribution of these products. We need our local officials to partner with schools to identify the distributors who supply these drugs to students. Most importantly, we must encourage our families and neighbors to do the same thing and to continue until we get the protection for our children that they deserve.

I think I witnessed the sale of these products to a minor. How can I report this to the authorities?

Sale of any electronic nicotine delivery system to a person under age 21, whether a pen, a pod, or any other device, is illegal in the US. Other potential violations include distribution of free samples of vaping or tobacco products or illegal advertising and marketing of vaping as safer or less harmful than smoking without FDA approval.

There are several methods of reporting a potential violation. You can report by sending an email to CTPCompliance@FDA.hhs.gov or by calling the FDA Tobacco Call Center at 1-877-CTP-1373 (1-877-287-1373). You can also report your concerns to the FDA online at https://www.accessdata.fda.gov/scripts/ptvr/index.cfm or print out a paper form and mail it to them directly. Once received, the FDA will evaluate your report to determine if the activity is a violation of the Tobacco Control Act or other regulations.

You can also make a report to your local authorities using non-911 services. In Texas, you can call the Texas Comptroller's Office at 1-800-345-8647, which is responsible for helping young people educate themselves about state laws on e-cigarettes and vaping products. The Texas Comptroller's Office is also responsible for investigation of vaping and tobacco sales to minors, minors in possession of tobacco or vaping products, and suspected criminal activity involving vaping and tobacco.

How can I set up community town hall discussions at my local school to help raise awareness about vaping risks?

The first step to raising awareness about the teen vaping epidemic is to discuss it with the people closest to you.

The harmfulness of vaping is well documented, but the public knowledge of these facts is not common. When more parents and neighbors join the fight to stop teen vaping, you can take the next step and discuss your concerns with school administrators and teachers. Look to your school nurse or school counselors for assistance with setting up a school-based educational event or contact your local Parent-Teacher Organization or Parent Volunteer Organization to create your own.

What resources are out there that I can refer to for more vaping and tobacco education?

Visit these websites for more information about the true dangers of vaping and e-cigarette use. Nearly all of these guides are free to use, print, and reproduce for nonprofit purposes. Some are interactive guides that actively engage the reader.

- ASPIRE: A Smoking Prevention Interactive Experience. www.aspire2.mdanderson.org
- CATCH My Breath – A free training module on vaping, part of the U.S. Coordinated Approach to Child Health, a nicotine vaping prevention program. https://www.catch.org/bundles/23725
- Fort Bend Community Prevention Coalition's Hidden in Plain Sight Mock Bedroom Walkthrough YouTube video. https://qrco.de/bdqVxn
- Make Smoking History – The Dangers of Vaping. http://makesmokinghistory.org/dangers-of-vaping/
- "The Real Cost" E-Cigarette Prevention Campaign. www.fda.gov/tobacco-products/public-health-education/real-cost-campaign

- 2019 National Youth Tobacco Survey. https://www.fda.gov/tobacco-products/youth-and-tobacco/youth-tobacco-use-results-national-youth-tobacco-survey
- 2022 National Youth Tobacco Survey Infographic – free color posters and printouts that provide summary information about the 2022 NYT survey. https://digitalmedia.hhs.gov/tobacco/print_materials/CTP-229?locale=en
- Vaping and E-Cigarettes: A Toolkit for Working with Youth (FDA). https://digitalmedia.hhs.gov/tobacco/print_materials/CTP-218
- FDA Sponsored Education Materials by Scholastic. http://www.scholastic.com/youthvapingrisks/
- Smokefree.gov – Tools and Tips to help you stop smoking. www.smokefree.gov
- FDA Safety Reporting Portal. www.safetyreporting.hhs.gov
- Truth Initiative – Become an Ex. https://www.becomeanex.org/
- Quiz on Hidden Vaping Devices – https://www.khou.com/article/news/health/vaping/hidden-vaping-devices/285-89df1874-8cf2-43f7-9c62-26bc044abbde
- E-Cigarettes and Vaping, a Texas Department of State Health Services website. https://www.dshs.texas.gov/tobacco/about-tobacco-use-control/e-cigarettes

Chapter 6

VAPING VOCABULARY GUIDE AND DRUG EMOJI DECODER

Every generation develops its own slang to communicate with each other. When it comes to drug slang, Gen Z is the master of emojis. An emoji is a pictogram or smiley face graphic used in text or other electronic messages to add emotional context or other information missing from plain text language. Emoji usage has become so popular because it can easily conceal conversations about the use and sale of drugs. The multiple meanings of images allow for plausible deniability while still communicating clearly to the intended targets. A transaction on cashless apps or social media may look completely harmless, but in reality, it might be a payment for purchasing drugs or other illegal substances.

Emojis or symbols are used to conceal details of the conversation from parents or general surveillance like social media platform administrators who use filter programs that search for certain keywords. The secret emoji language may also be used by illegal e-commerce sites to post drugs for sale without leaving hard evidence of drugs for sale to alert the authorities. These type of web postings with double meanings are making it easy for people to shop for drugs on their smart devices. Using emojis alone doesn't indicate drug use, but the DEA says that they are an indicator along with other warning signs.

DRUG DEALERS & ADVERTISEMENTS

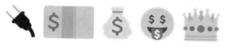

Dealers and distributors will often be called the plug and use the plug emoji. Other signals for drugs for sale include a stack of cash, a moneybag, the dollar sign smiley, and a crown symbol.

Here are some examples of emojis commonly used to represent drugs with their associated meanings:

MARIJUANA/WEED/CANNABIS

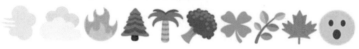

There are several icons that represent marijuana in emoji language. Be on the lookout for a puff of smoke, a cloud, a flame icon, a pine tree, a palm tree, broccoli, a four-leaf clover, a tree branch, a red maple leaf, and a surprised face emoji.

COCAINE/COKE

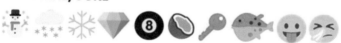

The emojis that represent cocaine include a snowman, a snowstorm or a snowy cloud, a snowflake, a blue diamond, an 8-ball, a coconut, a brown key, a blowfish, a smiley with tongue out, and a sneezing smiley face.

Although most cough syrup is available without a prescription, the cough syrup that contains codeine and other controlled substances are popular with drug users. Look for a purple crystal ball, a cluster of grapes, a purple heart, or a baby bottle.

COUGH SYRUP   **CRYSTAL METH**

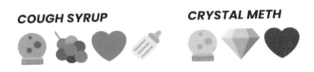

Methamphetamine, or crystal meth, is represented by a blue crystal ball, a blue diamond, or a blue heart emoji. Narcotics like Percocet, Oxycodone/Oxycontin, Codeine, and Hydrocodone are represented with the following emojis: a blue square with the letter P inside, a blue circle, a pill emoji, and a banana icon.

ADDERALL   **UNIVERSAL FOR ANY DRUG**

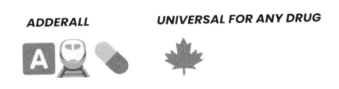

Adderall is a prescription drug stimulant used to treat attention deficit disorder (ADD) and attention deficit hyperactivity disorder (ADHD). It has a street name "A-train" and the letter A next to a train is often used to represent it. The pill emoji is used for many drugs of abuse that come in pill form. The red maple leaf is also used to represent many different drugs depending on the context of the situation.

PERCOCET/OXYCODONE   **XANAX/XANS**

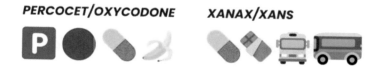

Xanax (Alprazolam), or the other benzodiazepines like Ativan (Lorazepam), is another prescription drug that is often abused. Its proper use is to treat anxiety. It can be represented with a pill emoji, a candy bar emoji, or a bus emoji.

HIGH POTENCY   **LARGE BATCH**   **SHROOMS**

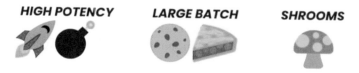

Psilocybin mushrooms, or shrooms, are a commonly used hallucinogenic drug of abuse. It grows naturally in tropic regions of the world, but it gets shipped all over. Look for mushroom emojis as the secret signal. The rocket ship and bomb emojis are used to signal if a particular item for sale is of high potency. The cookie and pie emojis often signal a large amount of supply is available for purchase.

Parents need to know about the secret lingo and emojis teens are using to find and obtain illegal drugs. Often, teens purchase drugs via popular social media platforms, hidden in plain sight. The Drug Enforcement Agency (DEA) also released "Emoji Drug Code: Decoded," a guide to educate parents, teachers, caregivers, and other authority figures to help everyone expose illegal drug use and identify the people selling them.

There is inherent value in the ability to discuss sensitive information in public without bystanders understanding the true nature of the discussion. The double meaning of drug language doesn't stop with emojis. The glossary that follows is a collection of new terminology and old language redefined to suit a new purpose.

4/20 or 4:20 or 420 - 420, 4:20, and 4/20, have become cultural slang synonymous with themes of marijuana and hashish consumption. April 20th is widely considered "National Marijuana Day," which, for many, is a "counterculture" holiday associated with the celebration and consumption of cannabis.

Acrolein – a hazardous chemical created when vegetable glycerin is heated; ingesting or inhaling it can cause cancer.

Amperage – the measure of energy flow of a vaporizer, also called "amps". The higher the amps, the more power is flowing to the heating element.

Analogs – a slang term that refers to traditional cigarettes.

Aqueous Glycerin – a mixture of vegetable glycerin and deionized water that makes a thinner fluid to make it easier to wick.

Atomizer – the component of a vape pen that delivers heat to turn vape juice into an aerosol or smoke form.

BDC/BCC – Bottom Dual-coil Clearomizer and Bottom Coil Clearomizer, both are heating elements, the part of the vaporizer that delivers heat.

Blunt – a rolled marijuana cigar where crushed cannabis is wrapped into a tobacco leaf paper.

Bong – an apparatus usually made of glass of plastic used as a filtration device generally for smoking cannabis, tobacco, or other herbal substances.

Cannabis – another name for the marijuana plant, but also can refer to the drug products derived from marijuana.

Cannabidiol (CBD) – a component of marijuana that has healing properties without the "high."

Carcinogen – a chemical or compound that can cause cancer.

Cartomizer – a vaping device that combines the vaping cartridge and atomizer, usually disposable.

Clearomizer – a cartomizer with a clear tank to view the e-liquid, usually reusable.

Coil – the part of the atomizer that makes contact with and heats up the e-liquid.

Dab (or Dabs) – slang term for small concentrates of butane hash oil.

Dab City – a state of mind or state of consciousness that one enters after consuming several consecutive dabs.

Dabbing – the act of using a vaping device to inhale or consume a dab of concentrated hash oil.

Diacetyl – a synthetic flavoring compound, giving a rich buttery taste, but also linked to lung disease.

Doob Tube – a small, airtight plastic container used to hide the smell of vaping and marijuana products.

Draw – to puff or take a hit from a vape device.

Dripping – adding drops of e-liquid directly onto the atomizer to increase vape smoke quantity and flavor.

Drip Tip – the part of the vaporizer that goes in the mouth for inhaling.

Dual Coil – any atomizer, cartomizer, or clearomizer that features two coils to increase vape smoke production.

E-cigarette – an electronic cigarette is a small device that uses energy from a battery to activate a heating element to convert liquid nicotine to an aerosol.

Edibles – edibles are food items infused with marijuana or THC. Marijuana edibles have increasingly become more and more popular among young people. The THC within edibles takes longer for the body to absorb, producing effects that last longer than when THC is smoked or vaped.

E-Hookah – an electronic vaping device that can be attached to traditional hookah piping.

E-juice – liquid nicotine mixture used for vaping; also called e-liquid or vape juice.

ENDS – Electronic Nicotine Delivery System, the official FDA acronym for vaping products.

Grinder – a tool used to break down cannabis buds into smaller particles that can be rolled into a joint or blunt.

Hash oil – a wax-like substance containing highly concentrated levels of THC extracted from cannabis, sometimes as high as 70-90% THC. Competing cannabis products contain 10-12% THC.

Hashish – a dry compound made from marijuana leaves used for smoking marijuana in a pipe, bong, or joint.

Joint – a rolled marijuana cigarette, most often hand-rolled, and designed for smoking.

JUUL – a popular brand of vape pen; also, the name of the company that produces a specific type of vape pen.

Mod – a modified e-cigarette, customized or personalized.

Propylene Glycol – a synthetic liquid used in vape juice but also used in food and cosmetics. It is safe to eat, but not safe to inhale. When heated, it can change into a new chemical.

Propylene Oxide – a byproduct created when propylene glycol is heated, which increases risk of developing cancer when inhaled or ingested.

Silicosis - a chronic inflammatory respiratory disease that cannot be cured.

Sploof – a cylinder-shaped filtration device used to reduce the odor of exhaled smoke from marijuana or other drugs, often homemade from a paper towel roll and dryer sheets.

Stash – a specialized container with a hidden space or compartment that is designed to mimic the outer appearance of normal household items. These products are often marketed as diversion safes to store valuables by hiding them in plain sight, however many teens use them to store drugs.

Tetrahydrocannabinol (THC) – the active component of marijuana that causes the "high" sensation.

Throat Hit – slang term for the sensation when the cigarette smoke or vape smoke hits the back of the throat.

Vape Juice - liquid nicotine mixture used for vaping; also called e-liquid or e-juice.

Vape Pen – a vaping device that is shaped like a pen or similar long and skinny shape.

Vape Pod – a cartridge of liquid nicotine mixture used in vaping devices.

Vaper's Tongue – This describes the loss of tasting sensitivity after excessive vaping.

Vaping – inhaling aerosolized nicotine or vaporized THC through a compact vaping device.

Vegetable Glycerin - a sugary alcohol derived from plant oils used with liquid nicotine to make e-liquid.

Vitamin E Acetate – a clear solution containing vitamin E used to dilute THC vape liquid to create more liquid to sell and therefore maximize profit; when heated, VEA decomposes into a highly toxic gas.

Wick – the material that is wrapped around and pulled through the coil that soaks up e-liquid to deliver the liquid to the heating element that turns the liquid into an aerosol.

About the Authors

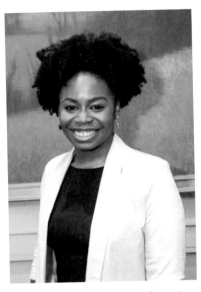

Lauren Ibekwe is a Coordinator for the Fort Bend Community Prevention Coalition. She serves a vital role in protecting the health and welfare of youth, families, and community members within Fort Bend County. Lauren has earned her master's degree in public health from the University of Texas Health Science Center – School of Public Health, Houston. She has an Advanced Certified Prevention Specialist (ACPS) certification issued by the Texas Certification Board. She uses her training to educate the public about the ease of access to drugs and alcohol, the underestimation of the risks of using, rising teen peer pressure, and other issues that increase adolescent substance use rates. In her free time, Lauren enjoys planning and hosting parties for family members and friends.

Payal Patani is the Director of the Fort Bend Community Prevention Coalition. She has served the Fort Bend Regional Council in this role since 2015. She holds a bachelor's degree in health education and Promotion from the University of Houston. She has also earned an Advanced Certified Prevention Specialist (ACPS) certification issued by the 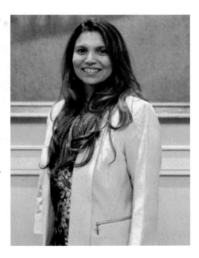 *Texas Certification Board. Payal is recognized as a leader at the local, regional, state, national, and institutional levels for her ability to prevent and reduce drug and alcohol use among youth and young adults. Her leadership led to the coalition being recognized by the Office of National Drug Control Policy for outstanding collaborative efforts in preventing substance use among youth. She is married to her wonderful husband, Hiren Patani, and they both enjoy raising their son, Dheyvir Patani.*

Dr. Uzo Odili is a first-generation Nigerian-American, whose parents immigrated into the US for higher education, in search of a better life for their future family. Born in Houston, Texas, he attended Bellaire High School where he became a National Merit Scholar. He then attended the Honors College at the University of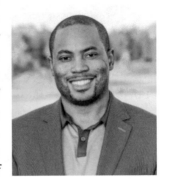

Houston and graduated Magna Cum Laude with a Bachelor of Science in Mathematics and a Bachelor of Science in Biology. He then earned his Doctor of Medicine Degree from the UT Houston Medical School before interning in General Surgery, then specializing in Family Medicine. He currently practices both Urgent Care medicine and Emergency Medicine in the greater Houston area and serves as the Medical Director at Apex Urgent Care Clinics in Katy, Richmond, and Cypress. In 2018, he was awarded a Top Doctor Award in Emergency Medicine by Houstonia Magazine. In 2019, he became a medical contributor to the Fort Bend Community Prevention Coalition and volunteers as a guest speaker for community town hall discussions to raise awareness about teen drug use. In 2020, he authored Vaping 101: A Q&A Guide for Parents and Teachers to provide fact-based advice on how to keep teens safe from the dangers of vaping. In 2021, he partnered with Mr. Organik, an entrepreneur and motivational speaker, to write Free Yourself, the Organik Guide to Financial Freedom, a book full of informative financial strategies. He is married to his wonderful wife LaTisha, and they are proud parents of their four boys.

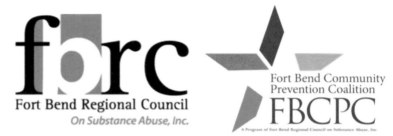

The Fort Bend Community Prevention Coalition is a program of the Fort Bend Regional Council on Substance Abuse, Inc. For over 45 years, Fort Bend Regional Council

has been providing families and individuals with substance abuse prevention, education, and treatment services they need for positive change for themselves and the community. The coalition is the council's population-focused youth prevention program. It unites many facets of a diverse community to collectively assess, identify and address local issues that contribute to substance use among youth and young adults. With over 40 active members, the coalition is a well-integrated, effective change agent. Its collective impact has increased capacity and advanced equity for prevention services within local infrastructures. These accomplishments support their mission, to prevent and reduce drug and alcohol use among youth and young adults by building healthy families, schools, and community environments.

Acknowledgements

Special thanks to Rashon Rose, the editor of this book. Your insight was instrumental in making sure that the book maintained a balanced perspective focused on delivering highly informative details while remaining easy-to-read. Thank you dearly for your help on this project and so many others over the years!

REFERENCES

[i] Huang J et al (2019) Vaping versus JUULing: how the extraordinary growth and marketing of JUUL transformed the US retail e-cigarette market. Tob Control 28(2):146–151

[ii] CDC Morbidity and Mortality Weekly Report. Notes from the Field: E-Cigarette Use Among Middle and High School Students – National Youth Tobacco Survey, United States, 2021. Weekly/October 1, 2021/70(39);1387-1389.
https://www.cdc.gov/mmwr/volumes/70/wr/mm7039a4.htm?s_cid=mm7039a4_w&utm_medium=email&utm_source=govdelivery

[iii] Park-Lee E, Ren C, Sawdey MD, et al. Notes from the Field: E-Cigarette Use Among Middle and High School Students — National Youth Tobacco Survey, United States, 2021. MMWR Morb Mortal Wkly Rep 2021; 70:1387–1389. DOI:
http://dx.doi.org/10.15585/mmwr.mm7039a4external icon

[iv] US FDA. Results from the Annual National Youth Tobacco Survey (2022). https://www.fda.gov/tobacco-products/youth-and-tobacco/results-annual-national-youth-tobacco-survey

[v] Wieslander, G; Norbäck, D; Lindgren, T. "Experimental exposure to propylene glycol mist in aviation emergency training: acute ocular and respiratory effects." *Occupational and Environmental Medicine* 58:10 649-655, 2001.

[vi] Henderson, TR; Clark, CR; Marshall, TC; Hanson, RL; & Hobbs, CH. "Heat degradation studies of solar heat transfer fluids," *Solar Energy*, 27, 121-128. 1981.

[vii] Wang H. T.; Hu Y.; Tong D.; Huang J.; Gu L.; Wu X. R.; Chung F. L.; Li G. M.; Tang M. S. Effect of carcinogenic acrolein on DNA repair and mutagenic susceptibility. J. Biol. Chem. 2012, 287, 12379–12386. 10.1074/jbc.M111.329623.

[viii] Varughese S, Teschke K, Brauer M, Chow Y, van Netten C, Kennedy SM. Effects of theatrical smokes and fogs on respiratory health in the entertainment industry. Am J Ind Med 47: 411–418, 2005. doi:10.1002/ajim.20151.

[ix] Williams M, Villarreal A, Bozhilov K, Lin S, Talbot P (2013) Metal and Silicate Particles Including Nanoparticles Are Present in Electronic Cigarette Cartomizer Fluid and Aerosol. PLoS ONE 8(3): e57987. https://doi.org/10.1371/journal.pone.0057987

[x] Conuel EJ, Chieng HC, Fantauzzi J, et al. Cannabinoid oil vaping associated lung injury and its radiographic appearance. Am J Med, (2020) 133:865-867

[xi] Chatham-Stephens K et al (2019) Characteristics of hospitalized and nonhospitalized patients in a nationwide outbreak of E-cigarette, or vaping, product use-associated lung injury - United States, November 2019. MMWR Morb Mortal Wkly Rep 68(46):1076–1080

[xii] Blount B. C., Karwowski M. P., Shields P. G., Morel-Espinosa M., Valentin-Blasini L., Gardner M., et al. (2019. b). Vitamin E Acetate in Bronchoalveolar-Lavage Fluid Associated with EVALI. N. Engl. J. Med. 10.1056/NEJMoa1916433

[xiii] Wu D, O'Shea DF (2020) Potential for release of pulmonary toxic ketene from vaping pyrolysis of vitamin E acetate. Proc Natl Acad Sci USA 117(12):6349–6355.

[xiv] Bhat TA et al (2020) An animal model of inhaled vitamin E acetate and EVALI-like lung injury. N Engl J Med

[xv] Environ Health Perspect. 2016 Jun;124(6):733-9. doi: 10.1289/ehp.1510185. Epub 2015 Dec 8.

[xvi] Curr Opin Pulm Med. 2016 Mar;22(2):158-64. doi: 10.1097/MCP.0000000000000250.

[xvii] Farsalinos K.E., Kistler K.A., Gillman G., Voudris V. Evaluation of electronic cigarette liquids and aerosol for the presence of selected inhalation toxins. Nicotine Tob. Res. 2015;17(2):168–174.

[xviii] Rubenstein ML et al. Adolescent Exposure to Toxic Volatile Organic Chemicals from E-Cigarettes. Pediatrics Apr 2018, 141 (4) e20173557; DOI: 10.1542/peds.2017-3557.

[xix] Wang H. T.; Hu Y.; Tong D.; Huang J.; Gu L.; Wu X. R.; Chung F. L.; Li G. M.; Tang M. S. Effect of carcinogenic acrolein on DNA repair and mutagenic susceptibility. J. Biol. Chem. 2012, 287, 12379–12386. 10.1074/jbc.M111.329623.

[xx] Henderson, TR; Clark, CR; Marshall, TC; Hanson, RL; & Hobbs, CH. "Heat degradation studies of solar heat transfer fluids," Solar Energy, 27, 121-128. 1981.

[xxi] Mohammadi L, Han DD, Springer ML, et al. Chronic E-Cigarette Use Impairs Endothelial Function on the Physiological and Cellular Levels. Arterioscler Thromb Vasc Biol. 2022 Nov;42(11):1333-1350. doi: 10.1161/ATVBAHA.121.317749. Epub 2022 Oct 26. PMID: 36288290; PMCID: PMC9625085.

[xxii] Huiliang Qiu, Hao Zhang, Daniel D. Han, et al. Increased vulnerability to atrial and ventricular arrhythmias caused by different types of inhaled tobacco or marijuana products. Heart Rhythm, Volume 20, Issue 1, 2023, Pages 76-86, ISSN 1547-5271,

[xxiii] US FDA. CTP Newsroom. Newly Signed Legislation Raises Federal Minimum Age of Sale of Tobacco Products to 21. https://www.fda.gov/tobacco-products/ctp-newsroom/newly-signed-legislation-raises-federal-minimum-age-sale-tobacco-products-21

[xxiv] Siegel MB, Tanwar KL, Wood KS. **Electronic cigarettes as a smoking-cessation: tool results from an online survey**. Am J Prev Med. 2011 Apr;40(4):472-5.

[xxv] Vaping in Texas Public Schools. https://www.tasb.org/services/legal-services/tasb-school-law-esource/students/documents/vaping-in-texas-public-schools.pdf

[xxvi] US Dept of Transportation. Proposed Rule on Smoking of Electronic Cigarettes on Aircraft. 14 CFR Part 252. Sep 15, 2011. RIN 2105-AE06.

[xxvii] US Dept of Housing and Urban Development. Rule Instituting Smoke-Free Housing. 24 CFR Parts 965 and 966. Nov 29, 2016. RIN 2577-AC97.

[xxviii] U.S. Department of Health and Human Services (USDHHS). A Report of the Surgeon General: How Tobacco Smoke Causes Disease. (2010)

[xxix] Jackler RK et al. Nicotine arms race: JUUL and the high-nicotine product market. Tob Control. 2019 Nov;28(6):623-628.

[xxx] Benowitz NL. Clinical pharmacology of inhaled drugs of abuse: implications in understanding nicotine dependence. Research Findings on Smoking of Abused Substances. NIDA Research Monograph 99. Chang CN, Hawks RL, editors. Rockville (MD): U.S. Department of Health and Human Services, Public Health Service, Alcohol, Drug Abuse, and Mental Health Administration, National Institute on Drug Abuse; 1990. pp. 12–29. DHHS Publication No. (ADM) 90-1690.

[xxxi] Dwyer JB, Broide RS, Leslie FM. Nicotine and brain development. Birth Defects Research Part C Embryo Today. 2008;84(1):30–44.

[xxxii] Chronic e-cigarette use impairs endothelial function on the physiological and cellular levels. Arteriosclerosis, Thrombosis, and Vascular Biology. DOI: 10.1161/ATVBAHA.121.317749

[xxxiii] Arain M, Haque M, Johal L, Mathur P, Nel W, Rais A, Sandhu R, Sharma S. Maturation of the adolescent brain. Neuropsychiatr Dis Treat. 2013;9:449-61. doi: 10.2147/NDT.S39776. Epub 2013 Apr 3. PMID: 23579318; PMCID: PMC3621648.

[xxxiv] Goriounova NA, Mansvelder HD. Short- and long-term consequences of nicotine exposure during adolescence for prefrontal cortex neuronal network function. Cold Spring Harb Perspect Med. 2012 Dec 1;2(12):a012120. doi: 10.1101/cshperspect.a012120. PMID: 22983224; PMCID: PMC3543069.

[xxxv] Quest Diagnostics. Nicotine and Cotinine, Urine. https://testdirectory.questdiagnostics.com/test/test-detail/90646/?cc=AMD

[xxxvi] National Center for Biotechnology Information. PubChem Database. Nicotine, CID=89594, https://pubchem.ncbi.nlm.nih.gov/compound/Nicotine)

[xxxvii] Soneji S , Barrington-Trimis JL , Wills TA , et al . Association between initial use of e-cigarettes and subsequent cigarette smoking among adolescents and young adults: a systematic review and meta-analysis. JAMA Pediatr 2017;171:788–97. doi:10.1001/jamapediatrics.2017.1488 pmid:http://www.ncbi.nlm.nih.gov/pubmed/28654986

[xxxviii] Hawes, M., Szenczy, A., Klein, D., Hajcak, G., & Nelson, B. (2022). Increases in depression and anxiety symptoms in adolescents and young adults during the COVID-19 pandemic. *Psychological Medicine, 52*(14), 3222-3230. doi:10.1017/S0033291720005358

[xxxix] Gotlib IH, Miller JG, Borchers LR, Coury SM, Costello LA, Garcia JM, Ho TC. Effects of the COVID-19 Pandemic on Mental Health and Brain Maturation in Adolescents: Implications for Analyzing Longitudinal Data. Biol Psychiatry Glob Open Sci. 2022 Dec 1. doi: 10.1016/j.bpsgos.2022.11.002.

Manufactured by Amazon.ca
Bolton, ON